Quality of life and older people

RETHINKING AGEING SERIES

Series editor: Brian Gearing
School of Health and Social Welfare
The Open University

'Open University Press' *Rethinking Ageing* series has yet to put a foot wrong and its latest editions are well up to standard . . . The series is fast becoming an essential part of the canon. If I ever win the lottery, I shall treat myself to the full set in hardback . . .'

Nursing Times

Current and forthcoming titles:
Miriam Bernard: **Promoting Health in Old Age**
Simon Biggs *et al.*: **Elder Abuse in Perspective**
Ken Blakemore and Margaret Boneham: **Age, Race and Ethnicity: A Comparative Approach**
John Bond and Lynne Corner: **Quality of Life and Older People**
Joanna Bornat (ed.): **Reminiscence Reviewed: Perspectives, Evaluations and Achievements**
Bill Bytheway: **Ageism**
Anthony Chiva and David F. Stears (eds): **Promoting the Health of Older People**
Maureen Crane: **Understanding Older Homeless People**
Mike Hepworth: **Stories of Ageing**
Frances Heywood *et al.*: **Housing and Home in Later Life**
Beverley Hughes: **Older People and Community Care: Critical Theory and Practice**
Tom Kitwood: **Dementia Reconsidered: The Person Comes First**
Eric Midwinter: **Pensioned Off: Retirement and Income Examined**
Sheila Peace *et al.*: **Re-evaluating Residential Care**
Moyra Sidell: **Health in Old Age: Myth, Mystery and Management**
Robert Slater: **The Psychology of Growing Old: Looking Forward**
John Vincent: **Politics, Power and Old Age**
Alan Walker and Tony Maltby: **Ageing Europe**
Alan Walker and Gerhard Naegele (eds): **The Politics of Old Age in Europe**

Quality of life and older people

JOHN BOND
and
LYNNE CORNER

OPEN UNIVERSITY PRESS

Open University Press
McGraw-Hill Education
McGraw-Hill House
Shoppenhangers Road
Maidenhead
Berkshire
England
SL6 2QL

email: enquiries@openup.co.uk
world wide web: www.openup.co.uk

and
Two Penn Plaza
New York
NY 10121-2289
USA

First published 2004

A catalogue record of this book is available from the British Library

ISBN 0 335 20872 X (pb)   0 335 20873 8 (hb)

Library of Congress Cataloging-in-Publication Data
CIP data applied for

Typeset by YHT Ltd, London
Printed in Great Britain by MPG Books Ltd, Bodmin, Cornwall

To the many anonymous older people who invited us into their
lives and freely told us their life stories

Contents

List of tables and figures

Series editor's preface

Quality of Life by John Bond and Lynne Corner is the nineteenth book to be published so far in the *Rethinking Ageing* series and it seems appropriate to locate it in the context of what has been achieved so far. The series was planned in the early 1990s, following the rapid growth in ageing populations in Britain and other countries that led to a dramatic increase in academic and professional interest in gerontology. In the 1970s and 1980s there was a steady increase in the publication of research studies which attempted to define and describe the characteristics and needs of older people. There were also a small number of theoretical attempts to reconceptualize the meaning of old age and to explore new ways in which we could think about ageing. By the early 1990s, however, a palpable gap had emerged between what was known about ageing by gerontologists and the very limited amount of information which was readily available to the growing number of people with a professional or personal interest in old age. The *Rethinking Ageing* series was conceived as a response to that 'knowledge gap'.

The first book to be published in the new series was *Age, Race and Ethnicity* by Ken Blakemore and Margaret Boneham. In the series editor's preface I set out the main aim of the *Rethinking Ageing* series which was to focus on a topic of current concern or interest in ageing (ageism, elder abuse, health in later life, dementia etc.) by addressing two fundamental questions: what is known about this topic? And what are the policy and practice implications of this knowledge? We wanted authors to provide a readable and stimulating review of current knowledge, but also to *rethink* their subject area by developing their own ideas in the light of their particular research and experience. We also believed it was essential that the books should be both scholarly *and* written in clear, non-technical language that would appeal equally to a broad range of students, academics and professionals with a common interest in ageing and age care.

The books published in this series have ranged broadly in subject matter – from ageism to reminiscence to community care to pensions to residential care. We have been very pleased that the response from individual readers and reviewers has been extremely positive towards almost all of the titles. The success of the series appears therefore to have justified its original aims. Now, well over a decade later, age and ageing are prominent topics in media and government policy debates. This reflects a new awareness of the demographic situation – by 2007 there will be more people over pensionable age than there will be children.[1] Paradoxically, however, the number of courses in social gerontology has actually decreased.[2]

So although there is more interest in ageing and old age than when we started the *Rethinking Ageing* series, there is still a need for the serious but accessible, topic-based books about ageing that it offers. However, having now addressed many of the established, mainstream subjects, we felt three years ago that it was time for the series to extend its subject matter to include emerging topics in ageing, as well as those whose importance have yet to be widely appreciated. Among the first books to reflect this policy were Maureen Crane's *Understanding Older Homeless People* and John Vincent's *Politics, Power and Old Age*. More recently, Mike Hepworth's *Stories of Ageing* was the first book by an author based in the UK to explore the potential of literary fiction as a gerontological resource. At the same time, we have continued to include topics of established interest as reflected in 2002 in *Housing and Home in Later Life* by Frances Heywood, Christine Oldman and Robin Means.

Quality of Life by Bond and Corner falls into both of these camps: the category of established topic in the sense of there being a long-standing and widespread interest; and that of emergent topic in so far as in the UK this subject has not been treated at book length in gerontology in a comprehensive, accessible way. There has long been a need for a volume which will explicate and rethink quality of life in a way which challenges established ideas. Since the inception of this series we have wanted to include a book on this important but complex issue and are now delighted to have the present volume by John Bond and Lynne Corner who have brought their own expertise and particular perspectives as highly experienced researchers both in gerontology and in health and social care to this volume.

Quality of life is now a familiar idea much discussed in the media and among the general public, although it may be defined variously by different people. The term 'quality of life' is however of fairly recent origin, dating back to the 1950s and 1960s, since when it seems to have been used increasingly in magazines and newspapers. At times, in advertisements for such products as cars, homes and holidays, it is treated as something which can be sold or marketed, equated with a certain lifestyle. But there is often a barely suppressed anxiety that materialism does not bring 'a good life'. There is indeed something elusive and difficult to pin down in the very notion of quality of life perhaps because of its philosophical dimension, and also because there are both subjective and objective aspects.

Within gerontology, quality of life is also a multidimensional concept, one with no fixed boundaries which has been of great interest to researchers for almost two decades. In 1990 Beverley Hughes published a groundbreaking and influential paper which mapped out eight dimensions as part of a conceptual model of quality of life and underlined its subjective and objective components.[3] As Bond and Corner say so appositely, there is now within social science an army of researchers pursuing this complex and confusing concept which has taken on 'the mantle of the Holy Grail', much of it relying rather dubiously on making 'objective' the subjective experience of the quality of life. The authors of this volume have been thinking about this topic for many years because they were unhappy with the definitions and interpretations of quality of life that many other social scientists, biomedical scientists, politicians and policy makers, were making. In rejecting this approach the authors bring their own research experience, including studies of people with dementia and a study of the private and public accounts of older people, to bear on this topic. Their book is thoroughly grounded in an extensive knowledge of the literature on gerontology as well as quality of life. One of its strengths is the way it grapples with the different dimensions and perspectives: with subjective and objective dimensions; and with positivistic and postmodern accounts.

The authors' approach to their subject is broad and eclectic. It includes older people's own descriptions of their quality of life; the experiences of growing older; aspects of the built environment and older people's living arrangements; statistical data on standards of living, family and social networks, and health and well-being; the meaning quality of life has to older people; gerontological theories; and key issues in the measurement of quality of life. Bond and Corner also provide an alternative framework for understanding quality of life and argue the need to rethink the way we use and operationalize the concept 'quality of life' in gerontological research and policy and practice.

This is both a broad-based and incisively written book which reviews what is known and rethinks its subject. It is a very welcome addition to the *Rethinking Ageing* series.

Brian Gearing

References
[1] *Guardian*, 29 May 1999.
[2] Bernard, M. *et al.* (1999) *Generations Review*, 9(3), September.
[3] Hughes, B. (1990) 'Quality of life', in S. M. Peace (ed.) *Researching Social Gerontology*, London: Sage Publications, pp. 46–58.

Copyright acknowledgements

We are grateful to the following for permission to reproduce copyright material: the author A. Bowling and Elsevier Inc. for Table 2.1; the author M. Farquhar and Elsevier Inc. for Table 2.2; the authors G. C. Wenger, R. Davies, S. Shahtahmasebi and A. Scott and Cambridge University Press for Table 2.3; the author M. Blaxter and Routledge for Figure 3.1; the Medical Research Council Cognitive Function and Ageing Study and Oxford University Press for Figure 3.2; the Controller of Her Majesty's Stationary Office for Tables 3.1–3.7; the author P. Towsend and Routledge for quotations from *The Family Life of Old People* and *The Last Refuge*.

We are also grateful to Dan Bolam for permission to reproduce photographic material.

Preface and acknowledgements

In 1999 we were invited by the series editor Brian Gearing to write this monograph. For a number of years we had been struggling with the way that 'quality of life' was being used in social gerontology and health services research. The desire to capture the essence of an older person's quality of life within a single independent variable dominates the post-positivist paradigm characteristic of much of the research endeavours of our fellow researchers and academics. An enormous research industry has developed to achieve this Holy Grail. For the last decade we have had a very productive working partnership in which we have been challenging the way quality of life in older people is researched. Our thinking has moved a long way since we first began to work together. The invitation to write this monograph provided us with a unique opportunity to collect together our arguments and to think through a number of conceptual, theoretical and methodological questions. This will be a continuous process but this monograph is a suitable milestone to celebrate. Our thanks to Brian Gearing for inviting us to do this and to Jacinta Evans and Rachel Gear at the Open University Press for their continuing encouragement and help.

The writing of this monograph would not have been possible without the stimulation from a wide range of colleagues around the world and the help and assistance of colleagues in Newcastle. We acknowledge the support of the Northern and Yorkshire NHS Executive and the Alzheimer's Society in England who respectively funded a postgraduate fellowship and a post-doctoral fellowship for Lynne. The studies completed as part of both fellowships involved a range of participants and we are particularly grateful to all those anonymous individuals who gave so freely of their time and who invited us into their lives and told us their life stories. We are grateful to the contribution of our colleagues in the ESRC Growing Older Programme, particularly Christina Victor, Sasha Scambler and Ann Bowling who have agreed to our using some of the primary as yet unpublished data from the loneliness project. The support of colleagues in the Centre for Health Services Research at the University of Newcastle was as always invaluable. It is invidious to mention individuals but special thanks to Claire Bamford, Jill Francis, Ruth Graham, Deborah Hutchings, Carl May, Elaine McColl, Tiago Moriera and Louise Robinson, who provided intellectual content and criticism. It would not have been possible to complete this book without the technical help of Barbara Ingman and Michael Norman who kept the computer technology up to scratch or the secretarial support of Cath Brennand, Maureen Craig, Linda Duckworth, Jan Legge and Beth Spiller who maintain the integrity of our bibliographic databases. Finally a very special thanks to Cath Brennand who as always made the final product come together in her usual quiet and efficient way. We are grateful to all our colleagues but responsibility for the content and interpretation of material rests, of course, with the authors.

The writing of books inevitably disrupts family lives and it would be remiss of us not to acknowledge this. But in all seriousness this endeavour would not have reached closure without the unending support of our spouses Senga Bond and Tony Morris.

1

What is quality of life?

On the whole, social scientists have failed to provide consistent and concise definitions of quality of life. The task is indeed problematic, for definitions of life quality are largely a matter of personal or group preferences; different people value different things.

(George and Bearon 1980: 1)

Introduction

The phrase 'quality of life' is now widely used, both in academic writing and everyday life. It is one of those taken-for-granted terms, of which we think we know the meaning. Although there will be some common understanding of what is meant by 'quality of life', we may use the term differently in our private and professional lives. We might anticipate considerable variation in its meaning for people of different age groups and cultural backgrounds as well as significant gender differences.

Quality of life is one of a number of social science concepts, which are regularly used in everyday life and have become part of the cultural and political vocabulary. Perhaps the classic example is that of class. Within most sociological theories of social stratification, class refers to the power relations between social groups, particularly in terms of economic power (Giddens and Birdsall 2001). Yet in everyday life it is used in a number of ways, most commonly to describe different social groups in terms of lifestyle and culture. Consequently it is also used pejoratively to stigmatize different social groups, for example the so-called 'underclass'. Thus in everyday life 'class' is used as a descriptive label rather than as an analytical concept. We may describe working-class people as economically less well-off than middle-class people but when invoking the vocabulary of the sociological theories of class, the nature of the power relation between these two groups only remains implicit.

A similar fate has befallen the concept 'quality of life'. Like 'class', 'quality of life' has been a part of social science theory for a number of years but in the last forty years it has slowly entered into the cultural and political vocabulary. In social science users of the concept belong to a broad church. Thus uses of the concept encompass the built, physical, economic and social environments, as well as the meaning of life to the individual and the subjective experience of life quality.

The purpose of this book is to examine the concept of 'quality of life' as used by social science researchers in studying ageing and the experience of later life from a critical gerontological perspective. We will provide a critical approach to the conceptualization and measurement of quality of life in social gerontology and health and social care research. We are not providing a sourcebook of methods or measures of quality of life since a number of these exist already (for example Bowling (1995a) and Carr *et al.* (2003)). But we will re-examine what we mean by quality of life in a postmodern world, by exploring the impact of continuous personal and societal changes on the lives of older people. In so doing we will draw on a wide range of studies which have reported on the experiences of older people and which in various ways present their quality of life.

The emergence of the concept of quality of life

Before attempting to understand what we mean by 'quality of life', we consider the emergence of the concept in the social science and gerontological literature. Two traditions have dominated the way quality of life has been conceptualized and measured within the social sciences: social indicators research and quality of life outcomes in health and social policy research. Both traditions are supported by a substantial social science research industry sustained by the continuing need of policy makers and politicians to evaluate 'quality of life'. The policy focus on quality of life in the European Union's research agenda and the work of the Foresight panels (Foresight Ageing Population Panel 2000) illustrates the continuing importance of the concept of quality of life to European public policy. Consequently both traditions have focused on issues of measurement rather than developing the necessary theory to underpin the concept and its operationalization in public policy.

Social indicators research developed in response to the growing dissatisfaction among policy makers with economic indicators such as Gross National Product (GNP) per capita as measures of societal importance and also to a rising awareness that despite economic prosperity and growth in standards of living in the post-World War II era, groups of the population continued to be dissatisfied with their social well-being (Carley 1981). The emergence of quality of life research in health and social care reflects the shift in medical preoccupation from the management of acute to chronic disease and the focus on morbidity rather than mortality as an outcome of medical intervention. The recognition of the importance of quality as well as quantity of life is captured by the World Health Organization's definition of health as 'a state of complete physical, mental and social wellbeing'. Although both these traditions were responding to different political, economic and social stimuli their parallel development has been important for the understanding of the quality of life of older people.

The term quality of life is a relatively recent term in the academic literature. It did not appear in the *International Encyclopaedia of Social Sciences* until 1968 and in *Index Medicus* until the mid-1970s. Life quality, however, was an implicit part of gerontological research in both Europe and North America for some time before. The British tradition emerged in the 1950s as part of the studies undertaken by the Institute of Community Studies (Townsend 1957, 1963; Young and Willmott 1957; Marris 1958; Townsend and Wedderburn 1965). This early work described the low level of material resources experienced by older people living in the East End of London during the postwar years and the poverty of the environment in which many older people lived. The tradition not only focused on the deprivation of urban postwar Britain but investigated the nature of urban communities, particularly the role that social networks and levels of social support played in determining a person's quality of life (Townsend 1957). Retirement, bereavement, loneliness and isolation were highlighted as important influences on older people's lives (Tunstall 1966; Townsend and Tunstall 1968). Much of this early work provided the framework for the development of the political economy perspective and the powerful theory of structured dependency (Townsend 1981) (see Chapter 5). The tradition has persisted to the present day through the writings of Chris Phillipson (Phillipson 1982, 1998; Laczko and Phillipson 1991) and Alan Walker (1980, 1981, 2000), among others, to provide a coherent understanding of later life and implicitly the quality of that life.

The American social gerontological tradition, which also emerged during the postwar period, focused more specifically on the subjective experience of later life. A core concept was life satisfaction, developed as part of disengagement theory (Cumming and Henry 1961) in the 1950s. A product of the dominant functionalist social science of the 1960s was the preoccupation with the measurement of life satisfaction (Neugarten *et al.* 1961) and subsequently 'quality of life' in American gerontological research, particularly clinical gerontology. This focus on the measurement of quality of life in older people reflects the dominant activity at the time which still dominates today: the measurement of the quality of life in health and illness. Within North America this has led to a highly productive industry for quality of life researchers and one which is now a global phenomenon. And, because of the preoccupation with health and ageing, it dominates our thinking about quality of life within social gerontology. It would be unfair to characterize the development of the concept in North America as without its critics. In a classic paper Jay Gubrium and Robert Lynott (1983) posed three key questions:

1 What is the image of life and satisfaction presented to subjects in the items of the five most commonly used scales and indices?
2 How might the image enter into the process of measurement?
3 How does the image compare with experiences of life and its satisfactions among older people revealed by studies of daily living?

These remain important questions and ones to which we return in Chapter 6.

Defining quality of life

It is not our intention to be typically ethnocentric in our approach to the topic of this book. In reviewing quality of life research it is evident that different studies have used widely different definitions and methods of assessing quality of life. These have been rooted in the cultures and taken-for-granted assumptions of policy makers and researchers. We do, however, need to provide some kind of framework in which to locate our discussion. From a critical social gerontology perspective two key principles have emerged. First, factors and criteria, which define a good quality of life for older people, are likely to apply equally to people from other age groups. Second, the experience of being an older person in contemporary society is determined as much by economic and social factors as by biological or individual characteristics. Thus, for example, in the context of chronic illness, quality of life is an individual experience which for older people will be influenced by their own general expectations and perceptions of older age and of living with ill health or disability.

Expert definitions

So what is quality of life? A useful starting point is Farquhar's (1994) classification of quality of life definitions. She distinguishes initially between expert definitions and lay definitions. Three major types of expert definitions are identified: global, component and focused definitions. Global definitions are rather general. For example Abrams (1973) defines the expression of quality of life as the degree of satisfaction or dissatisfaction felt by people with various aspects of their lives. Or, put more simply, quality of life is the provision of the 'necessary conditions for happiness and satisfaction' (McCall 1975). Component definitions emphasize the multidimensional nature of the concept and separate different dimensions of quality of life. George and Bearon (1980) identified four dimensions, two of which are 'objective' (general health and functional status; socio-economic status) and two of which are 'subjective' (life satisfaction, self-esteem). In contrast, Hughes (1990) highlights eight dimensions, or what she describes as 'constituent elements', as part of a conceptual model of quality of life (personal autonomy, expressed satisfaction, physical and mental well-being, socio-economic status, quality of the environment, purposeful activity, social integration and cultural factors). A modified version of this approach has been presented in relation to the quality of life of people with dementia (Bond 1999) and has been further adapted and is presented in Table 1.1 (p.6). The third type of expert definitions, focused definitions, centre on just one or two of these dimensions and tend to reflect the political or professional agendas of different disciplines. For example, within health services research, quality of life often focuses on health and functional status measures (Bowling 1996) and within health economics, on utility assessment (Torrance 1986).

Lay definitions

In recent years there has been a resurgence in the view that lay rather than expert definitions are more appropriate. A good example here is the way that the disability movement has redefined the meaning of disability from the perspective of people who are differently abled. Despite a long tradition in British social gerontology of listening to the voice of older people, there are few studies that have attempted to seek the perspective of older people about their quality of life. Claims are often made that the perspective of the other is being used, for example in the field of health status measurement (Fitzpatrick *et al.* 1998), but most approaches base this assertion on the fact that older people are providing the data. In this context study respondents will be simply acting 'as a passive *vessel of answers*' (Holstein and Gubrium 1995: 7). A particular issue here is the way that study respondents will structure their responses as either public or private views (Corner 1999). We explore further some of these theoretical and methodological challenges in Chapters 5 and 6.

Population surveys of older people rarely focus on the lay definition of quality of life. They use the standard social epidemiological framework encompassing expert definitions and concepts (see for example Townsend 1957; Hunt 1978b; Bury and Holme 1990; Bowling and Windsor 2001; Phillipson *et al.* 2001). Yet on those occasions where older people have been asked to describe their quality of life, 'older people can and do talk about their quality of life' (Farquhar 1994: 152). Older people talk about quality of life in different contexts but the important components (most frequently men-tioned) of a good quality of life are: family (children), social contacts, health, mobility/ability, material circumstances, activities, happiness, youthfulness and living environment (Farquhar 1994, 1995). Older people's assessments of their quality of life appear to be based on their expectations (Fisher 1992), which in turn are grounded in their life experiences and life biographies. In reporting their experiences older people made comparisons with the experience of their peers as well as within their own lives. 'They set their lives in context: the context of time' (Farquhar 1994: 153). In our experience the context of place and time, and the context in which older people are telling their life stories will influence the kinds and detail of experiences which are reported. Thus the perceived status of the listener, for example whether he/she is a health professional or social science university researcher, will have an important bearing on the kinds of stories and the details of life stories reported.

A conceptual model

Accepting that there are a number of caveats, existing research suggests that expert definitions, which use component definitions, are broadly in line with the reports of older people themselves. We can therefore think of no better starting point than to reflect on Beverley Hughes's account of the concept (Hughes 1990). Quality of life is a multidimensional concept, which has no clear or fixed boundaries. We have briefly seen that there is little agreement about what constitutes specific 'domains' of quality of life. Also it is clear that there are different perspectives on how to assess a 'high' or 'low' quality of life or who determines the relevance of constituent elements to different individuals.

Key domains

Many of the key domains of quality of life identified in social gerontological research reflect the demand for policy research and particularly the evaluation of the physical and social environments in which people live. It is therefore important to distinguish *quality of life* from *quality of care* (Bond and Bond 1987). To some extent the original list of domains generated by Hughes (1990) and her subsequent conceptual model of quality of life has been influenced by that agenda. Successful ageing (Baltes and Baltes 1990a) has not, until relatively recently, contributed enormously to our understanding of the concept. Table 1.1 (adapted from Hughes 1990) lists the key domains that reflect a research agenda, which includes positive as well as negative aspects of ageing.

Table 1.1   Domains relevant to the quality of life of older people

- *Subjective satisfaction*: global quality of life as assessed by individual older person.
- *Physical environmental factors*: standard of housing or institutional living arrangements, control over physical environment, access to facilities such as shops, public transport and leisure providers.
- *Social environmental factors*: family and social networks and support, levels of recreational activity and contact with statutory and voluntary organizations.
- *Socio-economic factors*: income and wealth, nutrition and overall standard of living.
- *Cultural factors*: age, gender, ethnic, religious and class background.
- *Health status factors*: physical well-being, functional ability and mental health.
- *Personality factors*: psychological well-being, morale, life satisfaction and happiness.
- *Personal autonomy factors*: ability to make choices, exercise control and negotiate own environment.

Subjective satisfaction

The most important domain of quality of life, if there is one, must be the overall satisfaction an individual has with life. This was a central part of the research done in the US over the last forty years (Neugarten *et al.* 1961; Palmore and Luikart 1972; Larson 1978; Campbell 1981; Chipperfield and Havens 2001) and has also been important in Britain (Hall 1976). The methods used to assess subjective satisfaction, however, have come under close scrutiny over the years and there remains considerable debate about what is being measured (Gubrium and Lynott 1983).

Physical environmental factors

The standard of the physical environment has been a significant factor in quality of life research. Housing quality has been judged by occupancy levels, the presence or absence of basic amenities such as indoor WC and hot running water, the presence of central heating in some or all rooms, as well as the general condition and state of disrepair of the building (Bond 1993b). It is noticeable how indicators of the physical environment have changed over the last fifty years, reflecting the relative improvement of housing stock since the 1950s. Similarly, the physical environment of institutional facilities such as nursing or residential homes have been judged by the proportion of single or multiple occupancy rooms, the nature of communal rooms, access for people with disabilities and again the physical condition of the building (Bond 1993b). The physical proximity of both housing and institutional facilities in relation to other community facilities such as shops and recreational facilities has always been seen as significant. But increasingly control over the physical environment has become an important standard of the quality of physical environments (Wagner 1988), reflecting once again the relative values of policy makers and society over time.

Social environmental factors

Family and social support networks have remained fundamental aspects of the social environment from the early community studies to the current day (Wenger 1996). This reflects not only the importance of the family and social networks in our social structure but also the policy maker's preoccupation with community care (DHSS 1983a). Apart from the family and social networks, levels of recreational activity and social participation (including paid and unpaid work) and the availability of formal and informal services have been widely accepted as important indicators of the quality of the social environment (Willcocks *et al.* 1987; Allen *et al.* 1992; Allen and Perkins 1995).

Socio-economic factors

Given the hegemony of the globalized consumer culture and the response of individuals to that culture, income and wealth are seen as *the* key factors influencing quality of life. In absolute terms the list of the basic essentials of everyday life is increasing. Adequate cover, nutrition and warmth are taken for granted. Inequalities in the overall standard of living continue to dominate academic and political debate. Relative poverty (Townsend 1970) and relative deprivation (Runciman 1966) remain important factors in a person's quality of life.

Cultural factors

In the social sciences we tend to recognize the presence of cultural differences resulting from the social status attributed to an individual's age, gender, class position, ethnic background or religious preference. When conceptualizing quality of life these factors are frequently treated as homogeneous but the reality is that there is often as much individual difference *within* social or cultural groups as there is *between* different social or cultural groups.

Health status factors

Later life is often characterized as one of sickness and infirmity. It is also, almost by definition, about the only certainty in life: death. It is therefore not surprising that health status continues to be treated by gerontologists as a very important factor in quality of life. Physical well-being, functional ability and mental health (Gurland and Katz 1992; Mroczek and Kolarz 1998) have all been shown to be associated with quality of life.

Personality factors

An individual's personality and psychological make-up are often associated directly with mental health but also function indirectly to influence quality of life. Studies have investigated quality of life in terms of psychological well-being, morale, life satisfaction and happiness (George 1979). But perhaps the most important personality factor to quality of life is a person's sense of self and personal identity (Taylor 1989).

Personal autonomy factors

Linked to personality factors but dependent also on the social and physical environments are personal autonomy factors such as the ability to make one's own choices, the ability to exercise control and the ability to control or negotiate one's own physical or social environment (Allen *et al.* 1992).

Quality of life as a relative concept

Apart from the ontological debate about the constituent elements of quality of life we have already hinted at two other key issues, namely how we define levels of quality in life and from whose perspective. The two are interlinked. Our dominant persuasion is to 'take the perspective of the other' and hence older people's perspectives on quality of life should, in our view, have precedence over experts. But from a societal perspective the views of experts in terms of, for example, resource allocation, will remain important. Therefore, although throughout this book we take the perspective of older people themselves, it is important to recognize that other perspectives cannot be ignored in the study of quality of life.

Determining the quality in life remains particularly problematic. We would probably all agree that a high quality of life is better than a low one. Yet it would be ethnocentric and inappropriate to make a judgement about the quality of life of other cultures, for example, Amazon Indians whose hunter-gatherer existence and low life expectancy is not something usually coveted by the majority of Europeans. (Of course, the concept of quality of life is very much a modernist concept and may not be one that exercises the thoughts of many people in traditional societies.) A simple solution to the definition of high and low quality would be to take only the perspective of individuals. How we each decide on what we mean by high or low quality of life would be an individual judgement. We can see that group consensus may evolve but within similar social groups there would always be individual pre-ferences. If we reduced our understanding of quality to the sum of individual subjective experiences there would be little point in investigating quality of life. Equally quality cannot be reduced to objective and absolute assumptions determined by experts. From a societal perspective we should also recognize that consensus is not achievable. (Of course it will still be of interest to investigate how individual older people and experts arrive at their particular definition of quality. A good research question from a constructionist per-spective would be about how 'quality' and 'quality of life' are socially constructed.)

Our preferred method of resolving the tensions between individual and societal perspectives on the one hand and objective and subjective definitions on the other hand is to define quality of life, like poverty and relative deprivation, as a relative concept. Such a concept must be grounded in theoretical constructions of ageing, something we return to in Chapter 5. Equally from a societal perspective it must be a concept that is measurable and have meaning for individuals within different social groups. We explore issues of measurement in Chapter 6. But what do we mean, then, when we describe quality of life as a relative concept? It is not simply one of individuals having different expectations of life, although this would be an element of it. Equally it would be inappropriate to regard quality of life simply as an aspect of relative deprivation resultant on the maldistribution of economic and social resources. But as a starting point we would argue that the quality of life of individuals is relative to the historical, economic and social context in which they are situated and will be influenced by individual life experience. We would therefore not expect older people to define their quality of life in the same terms as younger generations. Likewise we would not expect older people with disabilities to use the same criteria when assessing their quality of life as those older people without disabilities. We would expect people of different cultures to view quality of life in different ways. By using 'quality of life' in relative terms we are free in the following chapters to examine the concept from a number of perspectives and to ground the concept within a number of specific theoretical contexts.

This book comprises a further six chapters. In Chapter 2 we focus on how older people describe their own quality of life, situating their accounts within the context in which they are constructed. We draw on both explicit and implicit accounts. Chapter 3 summarizes some of the experiences of growing older in contemporary multicultural society. The chapter highlights aspects of the built environment and the living arrangements of older people. Data on standards of living, family and social networks and health and well-being are presented.

What is the meaning of quality of life to older people and how is it pre-sented by the arts and the media? Chapter 4 highlights the enormous variability in the experiences of older people and focuses on the meaning that quality of life has to older people. It also contrasts the different ways that the arts and the media have explicitly represented quality of life in older people.

How much do existing social gerontological theories reflect the concerns and interests of older people? Chapter 5 evaluates some of the key theories that could be used to explain the quality of later life. The chapter explores institutionalized ageism and structured dependency theory, and social participation and theories of productive ageing. It also examines the importance of self-esteem and other social psychological constructs that mediate the everyday experience of the social world.

How should quality of life be assessed in gerontological research? Chapter 6 reviews the key issues in the measurement of quality of life drawing on the large literature and experience from the health field. It will compare different methods used routinely in research and discuss the importance of gaining the perspective of the older person.

In our final chapter we bring together key issues from the previous six chapters and present an alternative approach to quality of life and older people. We will describe a framework for understanding quality of life that suggests the meaning that individuals give to their quality of life is probably determined by their life context: by the political, economic and cultural influences of the society in which they live; by individual lived experience across the life course; by their current expectations, attitudes and values and by the context in which the individuals reflectively provide this account. We argue for the need to rethink the way we use the concept 'quality of life' in gerontological research, policy and practice and suggest how the concept might be used more effectively.

2

Talking about quality of life

It doesn't matter how old you are, it's how you feel, isn't it?
(Thompson *et al.* 1991: 107)

We commence our presentation of quality of life and older people by starting from the accounts of older people as reported in autobiography, fiction, history and research. This cannot of course be a systematic presentation since the selection of sources is very much driven by our own collections of writings and the more obvious texts appearing in gerontological books and journals, and the analysis will be through the gaze of one young and one not so young social gerontologist.

In reflecting on the accounts of older people about quality of life we cannot avoid discussing what we mean by later life, older people and old age. As individuals, we agree very much with the Study participant cited at the head of this chapter and we suspect that this would be a widely shared view. The corollary to this statement, however, is probably 'It does not matter how old you feel, it's how old other people view you'! The way that age has been socially constructed within western cultures influences the way others view us, the way we respond and interact with others and consequently the way we are likely to feel about our own age. We live in a culture when every birthday is a further milestone along the life course. Specific birthdays are major milestones and imbued with symbolic significance: at 13 one becomes a teenager; at 16 one can get married and smoke; at 17 one can drive a car; at 18 one can consume alcohol and vote. By 30 we are already 'over the hill'; 40 is almost past it; at 50 old age looms; at 60/65 we can get the pension; at 80 we are 'definitely old'. These chronological landmarks are social constructions. Of course Shakespeare in *As You Like It* summed up, perhaps better than any one, the stereotypical social stages of the life course in his account of the seven ages of man (and woman):

All the world's a stage,
And all the men and women merely players:
They have their exits and their entrances;
And one man in his time plays many parts,
His acts being seven ages. At first the infant,
Mewling and puking in the nurse's arms.
And then the whining school boy, with his satchel,
And shining morning face, creeping like snail
Unwillingly to school. And then the lover,
Sighing like furnace, with a woeful ballad
Made to his mistress' eyebrow. Then a soldier,
Full of strange oaths, and bearded like the pard,
Jealous in honour, sudden and quick in quarrel,
Seeking the bubble reputation
Even in the cannon's mouth. And then the justice,
In fair round belly with good capon lin'd,
With eyes severe, and beard of formal cut,
Full of wise saws and modern instances;
And so he plays his part. The sixth age shifts
Into the lean and slipper'd pantaloon,
With spectacles on nose and pouch on side,
His youthful hose will sav'd a world too wide
For his shrunk shank; and his big manly voice,
Turning again towards childish treble, pipes
And whistles in his sound. Last scene of all,
That ends this strange eventful history,
Is second childishness, and mere oblivion,
Sans teeth, sans eyes, sans taste, sans everything.
(William Shakespeare, *As You Like It*. Act II, Scene VII)

But of course for social scientists what is of interest is not an individual's chronological age. Our concern is with the criteria used in everyday life that determine who is to be labelled 'young', 'middle-aged' or 'elderly', or who may be categorized as older adults, older people, people in the third age, people in the fourth age or deep old age. These criteria will be constructed within the context of particular cultural values and expectations. Of course within different cultures and historical periods each of these labels infer different consequences. It is generally believed that older people in traditional societies were venerated because they were social repositories of wisdom, custom and, in most traditional societies, property rights. But one reason why older people were better appreciated in traditional societies and pre-industrial Britain is that there were fewer of them (Laslett 1977). This contrasts with our postmodern world where youthfulness represents personal and aesthetic value and where the increasing numbers of older people no longer economically active are stigmatized as a burden on younger generations and experience the ageist behaviour of others.

As critical gerontologists who embrace many of the ideas of the political economy perspective, symbolic interactionism and phenomenology we would leave the definition of age categories to the important actors on our research stage. But this makes things complex for both us as authors and you as the reader, since we will spend the whole time avoiding the use of stereotypical everyday terms to describe various socially constructed stages of the life course. We therefore offer the following working taxonomy of terms along with our criteria for their use based on our cultural values and expectations. We add the caveat that no one individual will fit our categories precisely since we observe that older people represent a very diverse group of individuals. They come from a variety of backgrounds and cultures and throughout their personal life courses will have experienced many different events and social relationships.

Pensioners or people of retirement age

We try to avoid using these two related phrases because they tell us little more than using chronological age as the definition of old age. But historically pensioners have been a synonym for advanced age. It conjures up a stereotype of an older man or woman aged 65 or over living on the poverty line on the state pension and usually with some kind of physical or mental infirmity. Until relatively recently this was the label used for administrative purposes and by politicians.

Older people

A useful phrase that describes older people in contrast to younger people. Of course, when we use it we are doing so as a shorthand and recognizing the heterogeneity of later life. Administratively, official government documents refer to older people or older adults as people aged 50 or over. Increasingly, of course, this in effect is the new definition of old age based on criteria of being economically active, reflecting the decline in economic activity during the last quarter of the twentieth century of people aged 50 or over.

Third agers

People of the third age are increasingly labelled as third agers. The Third Age was a category fairly recently identified by Laslett (1987) and based on chronological age relative to life expectancy. In this taxonomy there exist just four ages of the life course. The First Age is used to describe an era of dependence, socialization, immaturity and education. The Second Age covers a large tranche of life and is generally associated with economic activity providing a period of independence, maturity and responsibility and, probably most importantly, earning. For Laslett (1987) the Third Age is an interlude when the goal of the individual life plan is realized until the onset of the Fourth Age. The Third Age offers the potential for greater individual agency and the opportunity to develop a distinct and fulfilling lifestyle separate from the world of work characteristic of the Second Age. Laslett (1987) emphasizes the separation of chronological age from this categorization of the life course. But the point of retirement is effectively the moment at which an individual enters the Third Age.

At its creation the concept of the Third Age was very much seen through a male and middle-class lens. It can be challenged as sexist and overtly moralistic. However, the term continues to have substantial currency and emerged as a useful concept over the last thirteen years of the twentieth century. Perhaps not surprisingly it has begun to be used in different ways. Three main ones have been identified, based on class, cohort and generational divisions within the social structure (Gilleard and Higgs 2002). Class has been an enduring feature of sociological analysis and class continues to influence the way the process of ageing is constructed (Phillipson 1982). From this traditional approach third agers became synonymous with WOOPies (well-off older persons) (Falkingham and Victor 1991) and 'well-off ageing' (Bury 1995). This is a relatively small proportion of retired people (usually men) who have greater wealth and larger incomes. The emergence of third-age WOOPies reflects the trend of an increasing disparity between the wealthiest and poorest people in all age groups (see Chapter 3).

An idea probably reflecting the demographic roots of the concept enumerated by Laslett (1996) is one that conceives third agers as being a distinct cohort of individuals. Thus in comparison with earlier cohorts of older people, current cohorts of people reaching retirement age have better life expectation and have had more favoured lifestyles including economic security. This approach still links third age to chronological age. This link is cut by the third approach based on Mannheim's (1952) ideas about generations, which includes not only a shared social location based on birth cohort but also a shared historical and socio-cultural location (Gilleard and Higgs 2002). For example the generation who were children during the Great Depression of the 1930s and survived the turmoil of World War II have very different values, attitudes and lifestyles to the 'baby boomers' born and brought up in the two decades after World War II. The strength of this approach is not simply that age (and being a third ager) is clearly distinguished from chronological age but that it recognizes the diversity of experience of older people at the beginning of the new millennium. Generational distinctions are important. With increasing social and technological change combined with the increase in disability-free life years will third agers not become an increasingly heterogeneous group? When this happens the concept of the Third Age will become redundant and we will need to find new ways to describe people from different generations!

Fourth agers

People in 'deep old age' and those in the Fourth Age may be known as fourth agers. The term provokes less negative connotations than others do, such as the 'frail elderly', although the need to distinguish fourth agers from other older people remains an ageist act (Bytheway 1995). Fourth agers will not necessarily share the same birth cohort, historical or socio-cultural location in the social structure. Their shared experience will be one of frailty, disability and social exclusion on the basis of disease and physical and cognitive impairments. We are not particularly happy with using this category since it perpetuates the medicalization of later life (Estes and Binney 1989) and we argue elsewhere the need for people with complex and severe disabilities to be treated as 'normal' human beings and for recognition of their personhood and citizenship (Bond 1999; Bond and Corner 2001). However, for the purpose of distinguishing from other categories of older people and in particular from third agers, selective use may be appropriate, although the danger remains that fourth agers may be treated in negative terms as were 'the elderly' or 'the aged' in earlier discourses on later life.

In summary we therefore use the following terms: older people, third agers and fourth agers. 'Older people' is used with a non-specific chronological age division to contrast with younger people and will include third agers and fourth agers. 'Third agers' is used to identify the current generation of older people who share the historical and socio-cultural experience of the second half of the twentieth century. 'Fourth agers' are those older people who are physically and psychologically dependent on others because of physical or mental incapacity.

Quality of life

What are the important elements of quality of life presented in the accounts of older people? There are a number, which emerge from the various sources that we have looked at: fiction, oral history, the classic community studies and contemporary ethnographies and case studies. Of course the methods used to elicit people's accounts will influence what issues they choose to focus on. We are thinking here not only about the way data are collected, whether by self-completed questionnaires, structured interviews or more open approaches as used in oral histories and qualitative studies, but also of the context in which studies are done. We have, for example, noticed that telling people where we come from affects their responses. In one study we only indicated to some participants that we were from the university. To others we informed them that we also worked in a Medical School. In this small qualitative study the latter group were more likely to talk first about their health and its effect on their quality of life than were those who only knew we were from the local university (Corner 1999).

Bowling *et al.* (Bowling 1995b, 1995c; Bowling and Windsor 2001) surveyed the adult population in 1993 as part of the Office for National Statistics (ONS) Omnibus Survey in Britain. Using social judgement theory (Brunswick 1956) and the approach to assessing quality of life developed by O'Boyle *et al.* (1989), Bowling invited survey respondents to nominate areas of their life that they thought were the most important in their current lives (both good and bad). Older respondents were most likely to mention freely their own health as the *first* most important thing in their lives, followed by their relationships with family or relatives and the health of another (close) person. Standard of living, social activities, spiritual or religious life, other relationships and environment were also rated as the first most important by a small number of respondents (Table 2.1). When responses relating to respondents' priority ranked areas 1–5 were combined, the most frequently mentioned area of life was own health, followed by relationships with family or relatives, finances/standard of living/housing, the health of close others and social life/leisure activities (Bowling 1995c, Table 2). Thus, different distributions were obtained depending on whether the analysis focused on priority ordering or frequency with which item was mentioned. Older respondents (aged 65 or over) gave similar responses to younger people but their priority was their own health. In addition a small proportion identified the local environment and religion and spiritual life as being important.

Table 2.1   Important areas of life for older people

Area of life	Most important %*	Proportion identifying any of areas listed %+
Own health	40	63
Family relationships	24	47
Health of close person	16	30
Standard of living	9	43
Social activities	2	21
Spiritual or religious	2	6
Other relationships	2	13
Environment	1	8
Other	4	–
Total	100	
Number of respondents	409	410

Notes: * Subject to rounding error.
+ Percentages add to more than 100% as this question was multicoded.
Sources: Bowling (1995b: Table 1; 1995c: Table 2)

Farquhar (1994, 1995) invited older people living in East London and Essex to talk about their quality of life as part of a longitudinal study investigating factors affecting successful survival of older people living at home (Bowling *et al.* 1997). The approach used in this study was to invite survey respondents to answer five unprompted open-ended questions about their quality of life. Answers to these questions were written down by the interviewer verbatim. In response to the question 'What things give your life quality?', family relationships, health, material circumstances (standard of living), activities and other social contacts were all reported (Table 2.2). Some respondents gave more than one item. References to the family usually meant their children. Activities included both activities in and outside the home such as going out to the park or watching television.

Like all surveys both these studies suffer from the difficulty of establishing differences between the public accounts of respondents and their undisclosed private accounts (Cornwell 1984; Corner 1999). However, the strength of this survey is the way that respondents were able freely to nominate areas of importance to them personally. The survey highlights the relative importance of self-nominated 'important areas of life' over so-called objective variables identified by researchers (Bowling and Windsor 2001). Farquhar's study suffers also from the same likely difficulty of reflecting the public accounts of respondents. Indeed it is difficult to conclude from both these studies which

Table 2.2 Things that give quality to the lives of older people*

	Sample 1 (85+ in 1987) %	Sample 2 (65–84 in 1989) %	Sample 3 (65–89 in 1989) %
Nothing	12	3	0
Family	34	40	49
Social activities	29	23	49
Other social contacts	25	23	21
Health	10	35	24
Material circumstances	10	23	21
Number	68	66	70

* Respondents gave more than one answer.
Source: Farquhar (1995: Table 4)

areas of life are the most important to respondents in their private accounts. They do suggest, however, that so-called subjective aspects of life be seen for the majority of older people as more important than 'objective' indicators of life quality.

Health and independence

That health is an important aspect of older people's lives cannot be disputed. Health predominates older people's conversations. It is often one of the first topics in conversations when two people of any age meet. We inevitably enquire when meeting others how they are. And if they are feeling less than normal one is likely to receive a detailed description of the signs and symptoms of their maladies. Hospital experiences are reported with great enthusiasm. Older people in order to define 'old age' also use health, in combination with incapacity and inability (Williams 1990; Thompson *et al.* 1991). So no wonder that health, both one's own health and the health of a significant other, is the leading nomination in some quality of life surveys.

Why is health so important to our perception of life quality? For many people ill health is a barrier to a successful old age and is the underlying cause of physical and psychological dependency. Ill health also reminds us of own inevitable mortality. Partly it is also due to the fear of physical and mental decline and becoming dependent on others for our basic needs. Thus in talking about health and illness we are probably overlooking other contributory factors to our quality of life that are less easily articulated or described in everyday life. In discussing health with older people Corner (1999) detected a number of factors that provided context and meaning to the participants' accounts of health. A sense of control and related feelings of self-worth, confidence, self-reliance and a sense of mastery emerged as aspects of health and illness. Important here were issues of autonomy, choice as well as control in the context of individual 'personhood' (Gergen and Davis 1985). Thus in order to understand quality of life and the importance of health we also need to consider the meaning of dependence and independence to older people. Control over day-to-day life events was found to be an important theme of conversations with older people. Who had control over day-to-day decisions? How this control was achieved and how it was maintained was central to how participants considered their everyday circumstances.

Self-confidence and a sense of personal control remain lifelong traits for many people, one that may only be modified by personal psychological work and significant life events. Heim (1990) considers the question of whether self-confidence increases or decreases with age. She suggests that physical confidence decreases in later life, particularly with increasingly impaired vision, hearing and more general physical movement. In contrast, social confidence increases. Heim (1990) suggests that older people are less concerned about what other people think and may play on their age to increase social acceptability of their behaviour. This strategy may reinforce ageism. Slater (1995) suggests that there is no evidence to support the idea that older individuals perceive a decrease in their sense of personal control as they age. For example, their coping strategies do not appear to use more passive approaches to problems. Neither are they less likely to try and master situations. Rather, individual differences in the sense of personal control remain across the life course. There may remain cohort differences, however, in the way that older people adjust to chronic illness and increasing disability. Younger generations are in general better educated and better education tends to be associated with a sense that more control is located within oneself (Slater 1995).

Social networks

The importance of family and kinship to quality of life has been generally recognized in social gerontological studies. That a high proportion of older people themselves nominate relationships with the family as the most important area of life and one of a small number of things that give life quality strengthens the importance of social support network theory in gerontological research. Unlike health, to which we found little reference in historical data, family and kinship has been extensively covered. From the work of the Cambridge Group for the History of Population and Social Structure under the directorship of the late Peter Laslett, we have a clear picture of the nature of family structures in Britain from the feudal society of medieval England, during the industrial revolution and the early years of the last century (Laslett 1977). Oral history has provided colourful accounts of life in the late nineteenth century and the pre-war years of the twentieth century (Blythe 1979; Roberts 1984, 1995; Thompson *et al.* 1991; Thompson 1992). These accounts suggest that when criticizing modern family life we look through rose-tinted glasses at the lives of older people in the past. As Laslett (1977) so eloquently argues:

> But if it is unjustifiable to think of the aged as being always neglected and condemned in our world, it is equally unjustifiable to assume that they were always cherished by their families and by their kin in the pre-industrial era. It is true that the fragmentary though suggestive evidence

which we shall cite indicates that the aged in pre-industrial England were more frequently to be found surrounded by their immediate family than is the case in the England of today. It is possible that they were given access to the families of their married offspring more readily than is now the case ... But we shall find that these circumstances can be persuasively accounted for without having to suppose that in the tra- ditional era in our country deliberate provision was made for the physical, emotional or economic needs of aged persons, aged relations or aged parents in a way which was in any sense superior to the provisions now being made by the children, the relatives and the friends of aged persons in our own day, not to speak of the elaborate machinery of an anxiously protective welfare state.

(Laslett 1977: 176–7)

Having presented his *fragmentary* data Laslett goes on to conclude:

The conclusion might be then that, as now, a place of your own, with help in the house, with access to your children, within reach of support, might have been what the elderly and the aged most wanted for themselves in the pre-industrial world. This was difficult to secure in traditional England for any but fairly substantial people. It must have been almost impossible in many other cultural areas of the world.

(Laslett 1977: 213)

The oral accounts collected by Ronald Blythe and described in *The View in Winter* (Blythe 1979) suggests that life for older people at the beginning of the twentieth century was no better. As the village district nurse, aged 84, put it:

Poor old things, poor old things! They weren't what they are now, I can tell you! Of course, they hadn't got the food, you know. They didn't get the living that they get these days. They say they're badly off now, but they're not, you know!

(Blythe 1979: 58)

And later she describes:

When I first came here in the twenties, lots of old people were neglected, really neglected. Even when they were still living with their families they would get dreadfully dirty ... And some of them were right tartars and families would long for them to die ... But other old people were gentle and good. Full of prayer I suppose.

(Blythe 1979: 59–60)

And in conclusion:

The old people came at the end of my day's work. It was maternity first and these old 'uns last. That was how it was arranged. They weren't only cottage people; I had the care of them in the houses, the rectory, the hall and such like. First mothers and babies, then my old men, waiting for me and looking out. Poor old things! Who remembers one of them now?

(Blythe 1979: 62)

Blythe's conversations with older people reflecting on the past provide a picture not dissimilar to today. Some families are close-knit and care for the older generation with respect, thoughtfulness and warmth while others would 'rather not know'. The value of oral history is the colour in the pictures of the past provided by those who were there. But some caution is needed since the individuals providing these pictures are selected by the author and to some extent are self-selected and may not offer a typical view. For stronger evidence we turn now to that provided by the classic community studies of older people in postwar Britain and recent contemporary accounts, some of which complement and some of which revisit them and contrast them to life in post-industrial Britain.

The classic studies of family life in postwar Britain (1940s and 1950s) were undertaken by Sheldon (1948) in Wolverhampton and Young and Willmott (1957) and Townsend (1957, 1963) in Bethnal Green in East London. Perhaps the most enduring picture painted by these studies is of older people embedded in kinship structures with strong family ties. As Townsend (1963) concludes:

> The general conclusion of this book is that if many of the processes and problems of ageing are to be understood, old people must be studied as members of families (which usually means extended families of three generations); and, if this is true, those concerned with social and health administration must, at every stage, treat old people as an inseparable part of a family group, which is more than a residential unit. They are not simply individuals, let alone 'cases' occupying beds or chairs. They are members of families and whether or not they are treated as such largely determines their security, their health, and their happiness.
>
> (Townsend 1963: 227)

The following extract is taken from one of three interview reports that Townsend reproduced in an Appendix. It relates to a point in the interview when a discussion about changes in family life takes place. This case example was provided as 'a classic example of the old living within a three-generation family setting':

> About former times, Mr Tilbury said, 'It was a hard time when I was young. We're happier now, we're more comfortable. We're happier together and more united. You've only got to look at these children. They're dressed up spick and span when they go to school. When **they** used to go to school there was hardly any of them with shoes on; you give me these people who say, "What about the good old days?" They were the bad old days. I don't want those days again. That's the truth. You never see children with a ha'porth of chips outside the pub these days. Families are more united than they were. You've only got to look at the babies in their prams. They're a picture. They used to put them in the bottom of an old chest of drawers. Or in the bottom of an old banana box. Things are a lot different now. And you don't see the rowing and fights like you used to.' And his wife interrupted saying, 'When we were first married, a woman stuck a head out of the window and looked down

at me, I was outside my house, and she said, "The Queen's dead. Can't you see I'm in mourning?" she said pointing at her eye. It was all swollen and black. Every Saturday night you used to see a bundle with somebody or other.' She looked at her husband and added, 'Me and him used to have a bundle. But we got used to ourselves now.' The husband said that 'husbands and wives get along better now. Her husband,' he said, looking at his daughter, 'wouldn't think twice of doing the wash- ing.' And Myra, the eleven-year-old granddaughter, said, 'Daddy does Mummy's hoovering sometimes too.' Her grandmother reproved her, saying, 'You shouldn't tell tales out of school.'

'We've been happy all our life. The only bad patches were when we lost our children. I lost a boy, he was only two months, with convul- sions.' She looked at her husband and said, 'Losing our children and your illnesses were the worst times.'

And when asked about loneliness:

No, we've always got plenty of people seeing us. We've always got our family. We've always been clinging together. I think families are more together than they used to be. Mind you, I don't say that's everyone. I don't class them what goes to pubs. We cling together.

(Townsend 1963: 289–91)

When respondents answer simple questions, they either give monosyllabic or complex ones. The respondents presented above fall into the latter camp and show how satisfaction with family life in the postwar years overlapped with issues about standard of living, relationships with neighbours and the wider physical, social and economic environment. Quality of life is not straightforward and the way it is described is far from simple. In another case Townsend describes a single woman who is familyless and objectively socially isolated; '... the most isolated yet encountered':

'I've never had any relatives in Bethnal Green and I've never seen any of them for more than twenty years. No, I'm not sorry I haven't any relatives in Bethnal Green.'

She said her biggest problem has been 'getting a living'. When I asked her what was the happiest time in her life she said, 'I've made myself happy at all times.'

She was most emphatic in saying that she was not lonely. 'I make my life. If I feel miserable I go out for a walk in the park.' She indicated in answer to other questions that she'd been used to a rather lonely life and therefore found it easier to amuse herself.

(Townsend 1963: 277)

Loneliness and isolation were one of the key issues identified in this study and one, which we return to below.

Has the nature of family relationships changed since this study was com- pleted and how does it reflect the world of older people fifty years on? Could the conclusion quoted above and the data on which it is based just be part of the optimism of the 1950s at a time when the British population were told that 'You've never had it so good'? One fact that has dramatically changed over the last fifty years is the living arrangements of older people. For the majority of older people nowadays the multigenerational households of the 1950s will rarely be experienced in later life but remain just a childhood memory. During the last half of the twentieth century older people have increasingly lived alone or with their spouses only (see Chapter 3: Table 3.2). Also, the nature of the local community environment, particularly in inner city areas like Bethnal Green, has become more 'hostile'. But these changes in the living arrangements of older people and the local environment have not changed the importance of family relations to older people at the beginning of the twenty-first century, as we have already seen.

Phillipson and colleagues (2001) revisited some of the areas studied in the community studies of the postwar era. There are a number of changes in the nature of social networks, which they observed. First, they found that the importance of the extended family had dwindled in the past fifty years. This is not to say that family relations were not still important. The immediate family clearly remains central to older people's lives. It provides a protective and emotional role to older people. The emotional closeness of the immediate family is highlighted by the following response from an elderly man living in Bethnal Green in 1995:

> Oh, I think that family is 100 per cent important. In every way because I mean for myself now this, I have only got one son right, there is peace of mind, I am under the weather, the wife had a very bad spell and so family life then was, it showed family life you know what I mean, it showed family life, everybody was prepared to, I mean at the drop of a hat they would be there, anything on the phone, I mean my son has got a car ... so you know family life is very, very important.
>
> (Phillipson *et al.* 2001: 64)

The second noticeable change was the nature of urban and inner city life and the impact that such change has on the nature of the family and older people in different communities. An important change has been the development of multicultural communities inside what were once relatively homogeneous areas. This trend is reflected in the diversity of languages spoken in inner city areas. Poverty, racism and dissatisfaction with the physical environment are aspects of quality of life in these communities. But equally there exists a diversity of cultural perspectives on quality of life. But older people in the three areas studied shared a perception of social exclusion and imprisonment in their own homes. For some it is features of the lifestyle and habits of some ethnic groups. For others it is the increasing fear and experience of crime and hostility due to racism. In such an environment it is not surprising that so much emphasis is placed on the importance of family relationships. For people from ethnic minorities such ties may be wider than the immediate family and perhaps analogous to the extended family of the working-class families of the 1950s.

I got mugged on the stairs. I used to like Bethnal Green but when I got mugged it turned me against it. There are too many Pakistanis around.
(Elderly widow)

I would rather live among white people ... there are very few here.
(Elderly married woman)

I am living surrounded by racist people, can't go out because of them. I don't feel safe. They don't like me to live here.
(Older married man)
(Phillipson *et al.* 2001: 98–9)

The changing nature of social networks is also highlighted in Wenger's longitudinal study (Wenger 1984, 1990; Burholt and Wenger 1998) of older people in rural North Wales, a very different setting to Bethnal Green. Although they are physically more dispersed, the importance of family relations to older people remains prominent.

In the 1950s relationships with friends and neighbours played an important role in the lives of older people but played second string to family and kin (Townsend 1957; Young and Willmott 1957), although relationships among 'housewives' and their neighbours and among men at their workplace were not insignificant. However, 'confidant' relationships normally remained within the family. With the decline in the extended family and greater emphasis on the immediate family, relationships with others have grown in significance, particularly among middle-class older women (Jerrome and Wenger 1999; Phillipson *et al.* 2001). However, among older people preference for confidants remains within the family (Wenger and Jerrome 1999).

Standards of living

We have already seen how in the postwar community studies poverty, housing circumstances and the process of retirement were intertwined with family life and people's perceptions of life quality. From the social indicator perspective levels of income, the quality of the local environment, the quality of housing and living arrangements are objective measures of quality of life. But from the perspectives of older people many of these objective indicators are irrelevant to the way they feel about their lives. For example, the school master in 'The Class of '09' when talking about the poverty of his childhood:

Things were hard but hard was normal. In any case I don't think that hard worries the young all that much. I was happy then, I am sure of that. Our poverty was dreadful and extreme, and nobody believed that it would ever go away. Now and then it rose up and struck at me personally and there was absolutely nothing that I could do about it. Or mother, and she had learnt ways of dealing with practically everything.
(Blythe 1979: 229)

But in those early years of the twentieth century the distribution of wealth was such that the majority of people were in the same kind of absolute poverty, a very different picture to a century later. Absolute poverty, the kind of extreme poverty that found children hungry and often shoeless, is almost now non-existent in the UK but relative poverty (Townsend 1970) is the experience of a significant minority of the population. Relative poverty is a concept that recognizes gross inequalities in the distribution of income and wealth in the population. For those individuals who experience relative poverty, it is their standard of living relative to their peers that sets them apart as being in poverty. However, some still experience a kind of absolute poverty, for example when they are unable to afford fuel to heat their homes adequately.

Older people in Bethnal Green at the end of the twentieth century, however, reflected the same kinds of concerns as their forbears forty years earlier. There were concerns about money and the feeling of living always close to the margin, as well as lacking the opportunities available to their better-off middle-class brethren. Respondents reported:

> Miss having money. I can't do what I want. I enjoy going down to the pub but I can't afford it, only at weekends.
>
> (Elderly married man)

> Not having things that other people have, like a car and holidays. I wanted to go to Clacton but the train fare was £15 each so we couldn't go.
>
> (Elderly married man)
> (Phillipson *et al.* 2001: 237)

Activity

Social activity covers a wide range and may or may not include doing things with others. In earlier times there was little opportunity for social activities, most of the day taken up by the effort of living. The exception here would be the small numbers of 'idle' rich, who spent a large part of their lives in activities for the purpose of entertaining themselves, so aptly illustrated in the various novels of Jane Austen. But for the majority life was continuous work and the need to fulfil the daily household chores. In 'The Valley' the miner's wife recalls her husband's question:

> He'd say, 'Can't you leave that till tomorrow?' and I'd say, 'Tomorrow will bring its own work.'
>
> (Blythe 1979: 216)

But for the average man and woman the routines of daily life have changed markedly throughout the twentieth century. Changing work practices, including shorter working hours and improved holiday and sickness entitlement, means that we all have more leisure time to fill. Family life has changed with the increase in women working and domestic life has been revolutionized by technology. These changes have led to an enormous difference in the lifestyles of older people after the world of work. As Phillipson *et al.* (2001) note, the lifestyle of older people in the 1950s was uniformly constructed:

Retirement, was, then, shaped for men by their talking in the street and in the pubs with other men; for women, it was the importance of home and street, in the company of other women (and children) within the family.

(Phillipson *et al.* 2001: 242)

But for third agers today the lifestyle is very different. First and foremost the length of life spent together by married couples is longer and couples do more together. Second, third agers have a wide range of activities. Phillipson *et al.* (2001: 242) document 139 different activities reported by respondents ranging from 'conventional social, sporting, hobby, educational and religious activities to the home computer buff, the stained-glass window maker, the radio ham, the political activist and the "people watcher" '. The most popular activities reported by older people (Phillipson *et al.* 2001) include: reading, gardening, watching television, walking, looking after the home, shopping, knitting, travelling, visiting the family and cooking. Although the engagement with social activities reduces slightly with age, undoubtedly because of ill health and infirmity, the diversity of activity confirms the changing lifestyle of third agers. There are important gender differences in the balance of activities with which men and women engage. Many women do not 'retire' since it remains a cultural expectation and norm that women will continue to take full responsibility for the unpaid work in the home (Bernard and Meade 1993; Skucha and Bernard 2000).

In research on loneliness (Scambler *et al.* 2002)[1] keeping active was seen as central to maintaining a good quality of life and preventing loneliness. Study participants stressed the importance of developing interests and hobbies that would allow them to fill their time productively and happily when they were no longer working. This was deemed important for people on their own, but was equally stressed by those who had stopped working and had to find other ways to spend their time: 'So many people used to say to me whatever you do don't retire. The secret is to keep interests' (Scambler *et al.* 2002: 9).

The significance of social activities for the life of older people demands greater clarification. Without making judgements about the relative value of different activities, say between watching television and gardening, in enhancing quality of life, it is useful to examine the impact of such activities and not make the assumption that having such interests increases life quality. Personally we would not consider our life to have much quality if all we did was to watch television, but for others it may bring considerable joy to their lives. For some gardening would be a great pleasure while for others it is just 'outdoor housework'. In the loneliness study gardening was more often a joy and one which engaged study participants the most. It was favoured by both men and women, no longer seen as just the province of men, as an activity which helped to maintain physical fitness, was creative, and was continually changing with the seasons and the uncertainty of the British climate.

I never get bored. I can always, well do the gardening or do some dec-
orating ... working in the garden, yes I can push myself in the garden
and it doesn't do any harm as long as I'm careful ... I mean until I retired
I never did anything. Well I mean I did a small amount of gardening but

I never knew a lot about it. Em . . . I suppose it has changed really. As I've learnt more about gardening I've got more interested in it.

(506;4;20)[2]

But the advantage of activities like gardening is the way it can develop into a social activity or indeed a particular third-age lifestyle. Gardening became a catalyst for other activities including membership of horticultural societies and the visiting of other gardens.

If we're at home we do like to go somewhere. We can go out and think we ought to do that, you know, maybe we go to the garden centre. This year we joined the horticultural society and so we've been to all sorts of places . . .

(702;4;47)

Loneliness

Loneliness or social isolation are rarely factors nominated by survey respondents in assessments of quality of life. This is partly because of the stigma of admitting to loneliness and partly because of the way questions are framed in surveys, which tend to focus on the important areas of life or factors that enhance a positive quality of life. It does, however, emerge as one aspect of later life that older adults approaching the age of retirement fear (Sarkisian *et al.* 2001).

Townsend (1957) made the simple distinction between social isolation and loneliness. Social isolation is an 'objective' assessment based on the number of social contacts with family and wider community. Loneliness is a subjective assessment based on 'an unwelcome feeling of lack or loss of companionship'. Modern discourses about loneliness present a more complex picture (Victor *et al.* 2000) but the power of Townsend's distinction is in its simplicity. We do not know the true extent of loneliness among different generations of older people. The stigma of loneliness militates against individuals expressing their private accounts so that much of our understanding of loneliness is based on survey data, which provide us with good estimates of loneliness as presented in respondents' public accounts. Townsend (1957) hints at some of the difficulties in his Bethnal Green study:

One difficulty had to be overcome. A few people liked to let their children think they were lonely so the latter would visit them as much as possible. This meant that they were inclined not to give an honest answer if children were present. In an early interview one married woman, asked whether she ever got lonely, said, 'Sometimes I do when they are all at work.' But she hesitated before answering and looked at her two married daughters, who were in the room. On a subsequent call, when the woman was alone, she told me she was 'never lonely really, but I like my children to call'.

(Townsend 1963: 195)

In the Loneliness study of ESRC Growing Older Programme (Scambler *et al.* 2002), we wanted to do two things. First to see whether the levels of loneliness reported in studies of earlier generations of older people were replicated at the end of the twentieth century and to investigate whether the risk factors or possible causes of loneliness had changed over fifty years. To do this we included the identical questions pioneered by Sheldon (1948), and used in the original studies, in an Office for National Statistics Omnibus Survey. The second thing we wanted to do was to investigate both the private and public accounts of older people. To do this we conducted a number of qualitative interviews with a selected sample of respondents in the Omnibus Survey.

The review on the prevalence of loneliness (Victor *et al.* 2000) suggests that the extent of loneliness in people aged 65 or over ranged from 5 per cent to 16 per cent with a median of 9–10 per cent (Sheldon 1948; Townsend 1957; Tunstall 1966; Townsend and Tunstall 1968; Hunt 1978a; Bond and Carstairs 1982; Wenger 1984; Jones *et al.* 1985; Qureshi and Walker 1989; Bowling and Farquhar 1991). Data from the Loneliness study of ESRC Growing Older Programme found that 9 per cent of respondents were always or often lonely, 37 per cent sometimes lonely and 54 per cent never lonely. These estimates are similar to earlier studies although there may be an indication that older people are now more willing to admit to being lonely sometimes, the proportion reporting being sometimes lonely increasing from about 20 per cent in the 1950s to nearer 40 per cent in 2000 (Victor *et al.* 2002).

With the objective of trying to ameliorate loneliness among older people a number of studies have been concerned with highlighting the risk factors for loneliness and identifying the causes of loneliness. Sheldon (1948) recognized that there seemed to be no single cause of severe loneliness (people who report that they are always or often lonely in community surveys). Townsend, summarizing Sheldon, concluded:

> Loneliness cannot be regarded as the simple direct result of social circumstances, but is rather an individual response to an external situation to which other old people may react quite differently. The main exception being when the death of a spouse was recent.
>
> (Townsend 1963: 195–6)

For Townsend (1973a, 1973b; Townsend and Tunstall 1968) loss or separation was a significant cause of loneliness and he introduced the concept of desolation to distinguish those older people who were profoundly lonely (and probably depressed) as a result of bereavement. There has been little attempt by contemporary gerontologists to explore these ideas further among current generations of older people. Much of the research has focused on identifying statistical correlates between a range of covariates and social isolation or loneliness. There exist no direct links between demographic, behavioural and social variables and social isolation and loneliness, but many similar factors appear to be associated with both (Wenger *et al.* 1996). One of the challenges to defining a consistent theory for understanding the causes of loneliness and isolation has been the different ways of defining these two concepts, inconsistency of interpretations between different studies and the lack of good longitudinal data. Existing data are therefore limited to reporting associations between demographic, behavioural and social variables and social isolation or loneliness. A summary of reported correlates of isolation and loneliness is shown in Table 2.3.

Table 2.3 Summary of reported correlates* of isolation and loneliness

	Isolation	Loneliness
Personal circumstances		
Age	X	X
Male sex	X	X
Widowhood	X	X
Singleness	X	X
Living alone	X	X
Childlessness	X	X
Resources		
Absence of friends		X
Poor health	X	X
Restricted mobility	X	X
Mortality	X	X
Mental illness	X	
Depression		X
Low morale	X	X
Working-class status	X	
Life events		
Admission to long-term care	X	X
Poor rehabilitation	X	
Retirement migration	X	X
Loss		X

* All statistical associations as shown in table are positive.

Source: Adapted from Wenger *et al.* (1996: Table 2)

In the Loneliness study of ESRC Growing Older Programme we identified 'risk factors' for loneliness and social isolation (Victor *et al.* 2004). 'Risk factors' for loneliness were grouped into categories: socio-economic, health resources, material resources, social resources and social networks. The relationship between each variable and the prevalence of loneliness was tested in order to identify 'peer group' patterns of loneliness. This analysis revealed that loneliness was most likely to be reported by specific groups of older people: people who were very old, women, those who were not married, those who lived alone, those lacking material resources (non-home or car owners), those without educational qualifications, those who were physically or mentally frail and those who spent long periods of time alone. No relationship was observed with levels of contact with family, friends or neighbours.

Clearly many of these factors are interrelated and to gain a more accurate picture a more detailed analysis was undertaken. Factors not independently associated with the outcome variable, loneliness, were eliminated. This exercise revealed that there were both factors that increased 'vulnerability' to loneliness and those that had a 'protective' effect. Greater vulnerability to loneliness was associated independently with six characteristics: not being married (with widowed people being most vulnerable), increased time spent alone, increased perception of loneliness over previous decade, poor health rating, health worse in old age than expected and mental morbidity (as measured by the General Health Questionnaire [GHQ-12]; Goldberg and Williams 1988). Two factors were independently associated with decreased likelihood of experiencing loneliness. These were advanced age and the possession of educational qualifications.

The experience of loneliness

To date statistical analysis of large surveys of different populations provide only minimal insight into the relationship between isolation or loneliness and quality of life. Although the ESRC Growing Older Programme gives contemporary estimates, by itself it gives little greater insight than the earlier community studies. On the other hand the qualitative interviews conducted as part of the ESRC Growing Older Programme provide greater insight into a number of issues. A key issue for the study is about the experience of loneliness. The public account of loneliness captured in the survey was found to be very similar to the range of surveys reported over the last fifty years. However, the private account captured during qualitative interviews began to present quite a different picture of the prevalence of loneliness. Predominantly participants were third agers, three-quarters (34 of 45) were aged between 65 and 79. Of 45 participants in the qualitative follow-up study only 7 (15 per cent) reported being 'always' or 'often lonely' at the time of the survey. But during the qualitative interviews 26 (58 per cent) reported being lonely and for a further 6 the investigator was confident that they were not able to report their feelings of loneliness.

What do older people mean when they talk about loneliness? Participants in the Loneliness study of ESRC Growing Older Programme qualitative interviews were asked to give their understanding. For them, there were three distinct ways of conceptualizing loneliness. First, it related to their social networks, particularly their family. Second, it was about the absence of personal and social resources such as immobility and the lack of finance. Third, loneliness was described as a state of mind; it was up to the individual. Over a third (17 of 44) of participants used a combination of the three to describe what loneliness meant to them.

The majority (32 of 44) of older people interviewed highlighted social network in their response. The key idea here is that loneliness is linked to the number of friends and relations that people have around them and the closeness of the relationships between members of the network. This fits in very well with Townsend's (1957) idea of a feeling of the lack of companionship and the general scientific view that loneliness results from an inadequate social network. The latter does not, however, quite square with the considerable literature, which shows that an inadequate social network is neither a necessary or sufficient characteristic of loneliness. Other factors are also important. But for the majority of participants the most important feature of an adequate social network was the presence of a confidant. The presence of a confidant has been found to protect against depression (Brown and Harris 1978) and in this study the loss of a confidant, particularly the loss of a long-term partner, was a major cause of loneliness:

> Loneliness ... It can almost be physical ... I've got everything but I haven't got enough. I ... er ... you can never replace a wife. You can never replace a partner. You can't turn it on and off like a tap. If you love someone for that many years, it's a very lonely life.
>
> (402;5;25)

For many, the loss of others of the same generation, siblings and friends, either through relocation or death, is influential in their understanding of loneliness:

> We've got a lot of friends gone abroad to live so they're sort of dwindling. But now we find that as you're getting older you're losing friends because we've lost two or three friends that have died recently, you know, and you don't make new ones.
>
> (701;4;18)

But as we have already seen, close contact with the extended family, particularly grandchildren, was also considered to be an extremely important factor in thwarting loneliness.

The loss or lack of resources in later life can take many forms and they can also accumulate and lead to a sense of loneliness, although usually in combination with one of the other two senses of the term. For example, one couple identified a combination of losses in their lives, financial losses and the loss of health:

> We get out when we can but we haven't got the money to do as much as we would like. That's why we moved up here. Because when we retired, we retired in 1990, I sold my business and it was let out and they went bust and we've lost all our extra pension. So we sold our house down there but we haven't got the money we should have had so it means we can only get out sometimes ... We used to play golf, but I don't think I could now in any case because of the arthritis, but we would have played up here, you know, if we'd come up before when we'd got the money. And there are a lot of other things that don't cost much.
>
> (601;3;13)

Loneliness has been described by some as 'a state of mind', the causes being solely attributable to the individual's ability to find ways of filling time and not being bored, happiness and contentment at spending time alone, the willingness to get up and make yourself do something and attitude of mind that allows you to go out and meet new people and make new friends. This perspective is summed up by the following comment from a participant in the ESRC Growing Older Programme:

> Well when I first came here I decided that it is the village and that if I wanted to sit indoors nobody was going to knock on my front door so I joined what they called the 'Trimley Wives' ... And through that I've met a lot of people and I've made a very good friend. She's 62 and we've

become quite good friends, and we go abroad together as well . . . But life is quite good and it's interesting. But if you want to sit indoors and don't go out the front door then nobody is going to make the effort to get to know you.

(305;3;34)

Spirituality and the meaning of life

Religion has played a central role in the structure of societies and in providing different perspectives on the meaning of life. Each of the world religions provides the basis of the core values and principles upon which contemporary life is founded. Yet the relevance of religion to individuals in the UK declined in the last half of the twentieth century (Coleman *et al.* 2002), although the vast majority of people around the world continue to believe in a God or universal spirit (Koenig 1993). For these individuals religion provides a meaning to life in terms of social integration and participation and a meaning of life in terms of the very reason for their existence. The decline in religiosity has not necessarily been accompanied by a decline in the search for the answer to the ultimate question of human kind: why do I exist? Historically little distinction was made between religion and spirituality (George *et al.* 2000) and it is only recently that these have come to be seen as two distinct but complementary ideas. The secularization of society and disillusionment with religious institutions is cited as contributory to the emergence of this distinction (Sheldrake 1992). Religion and spirituality share a focus on the sacred or divine, beliefs about the sacred, the effect of those beliefs on behaviour and practices used to maintain a sense of the sacred. But, while religion is strongly linked to powerful religious institutions, spirituality remains an immensely individual experience outside an institutional or collective context. The distinction often cited in the sociology of organizations between formal and informal organization has relevance here. The formal organization of most world religions, based on power and rationality, contrasts with the informal composition of spirituality grounded in personal autonomy, beliefs and sentiment.

Religious beliefs and spiritual behaviour are common among older people and appear to increase in frequency with age (Koenig 1993). In adversity older adults seek religious and spiritual solutions to their problems of health, loneliness or hopelessness. But for the devoutly religious, their faith remains a higher ascetic. In *The View in Winter* (Blythe 1979) Colonel Hardy from the Salvation Army reflects on being old:

I have to admit that I don't feel old and I do feel profoundly happy, but that's the way life has gone. I've led the religious life and it seems to have worked. Though it's not for me to say. Ours is an experimental faith, not just an intellectual one. Our religion is far more experimental than credal. I have had to apply it to such a succession of social changes in my lifetime that it had to be flexible. It should be flexible. Love is flexible. It winds round everything, I don't think that I ever thought about being old when I was being young! And I wouldn't want it – life –

all over again. Once is enough. Young people often say 'Would you like to be young again?' and don't really like it when you say no. I soften the blow. I say, 'Just think of all those years I should have been done out of heaven!'

(Blythe 1979: 311)

The clergyman's wife also exhibits devout religiosity in her reflections on dying:

I don't dread dying in my sleep but I do dread dying any other way. Mostly for the nuisance you know. And I don't dread being dead. My heavenly father has looked after me from the cradle and he won't stop at the grave. Through all my life he has taken care of me. Even if I went out like a candle, what is there to dread?

(Blythe 1979: 319)

Religion was an important part of British life prior to World War II. The oral history narratives reported by Thompson *et al.* (1991) are dotted with accounts of family bible readings and formal church attendance. For example 'a Stepney dairyman's daughter had to call every Sunday morning on the way to church, to read her grandfather a verse from the Bible' (Thompson *et al.* 1991: 80). Loss of a loved one in later life triggered spiritual behaviour. Koenig (1993) concludes that as times get harder religion takes on greater and greater importance, particularly for those growing older who must face declines in health and loss of companionship and independence. But recent data from the ESRC Growing Older Programme suggests that this trend observed in the US is not reproduced in the UK (Coleman *et al.* 2002). The qualitative data from the loneliness study is remarkable by the absence of accounts of religious and spiritual behaviour. Where religion was mentioned it focused mainly on religious affiliation and participation. Other domains including religious or spiritual values and those concerned with the meaning of life were noticeable by their absence. Spirituality was not a theme that emerged strongly within the data.

Religious and spiritual behaviour has been credited with improving health and personal well-being (Koenig 1993, 1995; McFadden 1999; George *et al.* 2000). But an exploratory qualitative case study of twenty-eight older bereaved spouses suggests that those with moderate beliefs may be at greater risk of depression (Coleman *et al.* 2002). One of the explanations suggested is the nature of moderate beliefs. Study participants were not necessarily members of churches and religious organizations. All eleven moderate believers provided indications of the unsatisfactory nature of their spiritual beliefs and its association with low perceived meaning in their lives. They question their faith and live in uncertainty about the future of life and life after death. In the UK, at least, the positive value of religious and spiritual behaviour appears more complex than the conclusions drawn from US studies. The spiritual turmoil experienced by some older people about their spiritual beliefs militates against perceptions of a positive overall quality of life.

Talking about life

The selected edited private accounts told by older people provide a rich description of older people's lives across the twentieth century. They both confirm and contradict the stereotypes we might hold based on the public accounts captured in surveys and structured interviews. For each individual different aspects of their lives are important to their quality of life. But over all there is a general consensus that own and others' health, family relationships and social networks, social activity, standard of living and spirituality are important elements in the experience of older people's lives. The relative importance to any one individual may change across the life course and within the context of time and space. There may be differences between the accounts of third agers and those who have reached 'deep old age' and between people from different social and cultural groups. In the next chapter we take a more social-indicator approach and report survey data of the social and material resources of older people. We will return to the accounts and stories of older people in Chapters 5 and 6 when we seek to provide an understanding to the theoretical and methodological issues surrounding quality of life and older people.

Notes

1. Study funded as part of ESRC Growing Older Programme. A full analysis of the study will be presented in Victor, Scambler and Bond (forthcoming) *The World of Older People*, Open University Press.
2. Unpublished data from the Loneliness study of ESRC Growing Older Programme. Numbers indicate [Transcript identifier; page number; line number].

3

Environment and quality of life

Older people are not a homogeneous group. Like the rest of the population there are differences in gender, 'race' and ethnicity, socio-economic group/social class, income/pensions, regional/local cultures and household and/or family structure.
                            (Joint Taskforce on Older People 2000: Box 1, p. 2)

In the previous chapter we reported the accounts of older people in which they describe their quality of life. We have argued that the way these accounts are formed will depend on the context of individual life biographies and self-identities. In this chapter we take a more traditional view of quality of life by exploring the physical and social environments in which older people live. We will also examine cultural, socio-economic and health status factors which influence the quality of older people's lives.

The physical environment

The vicissitudes of physical environments in which older people live reflects the diversity of experience of the wider population. One exception is the quality of long-term care institutions, where the majority of residents are older people (usually aged 80 or over). The urban and rural landscapes of Europe are forever changing. The last fifty years have seen substantial regeneration of some inner cities, a decline in many traditional industrial and manufacturing communities and crisis in the rural community. Changes in the built environment of communities has given us homogeneous ghetto-like housing estates for different socio-economic groups, the hegemony of out-of-town shopping centres, a decline in small towns and villages, and the development of new and traditional retirement areas. Official statistics fail to capture the reality of the broad physical environment in which we all live at the beginning of the twenty-first century. Photographic evidence, journalistic accounts and contemporary novels may provide a better perspective although these reflect the artists' and writers' choices of images to describe.

The homes of older people

In Britain, like other European countries, about 95 per cent of people aged 60 years or over live in private households (OPCS/GRO(S) 1993), although as people age they are likely to experience living in some kind of institution or communal establishment. Of older people living in private households about 5 per cent will live in some kind of sheltered accommodation with a warden and a further 5 per cent in sheltered accommodation without a warden (Bridgwood 2000: Table 7). The level of provision of sheltered housing in the UK is highest among members of the European Union. Scandinavian countries also have a significant provision but sheltered accommodation is practically non-existent in Austria, Greece, Spain and Portugal (Pacolet *et al.* 2000: Figure 3.10).

Over the last fifty years there has been a steady increase in owner-occupation in Britain. Until 1980 there was an equally steady increase in the provision of social housing at the expense of the privately rented sector (Boleat 1986), although there are substantial regional variations. Other member states within the European Union have a stronger tradition of owner-occupation and the private renting of housing. However, many states provide subsidies to citizens with low incomes (Pacolet *et al.* 2000). Trends in home ownership in Britain have been reflected in the experiences of older people. In 1980 47 per cent, in 1991 58 per cent and in 1998 68 per cent of households containing at least one person aged 65 or over were owner-occupier households (Bridgwood 2000: Table 5). About a third of the increase in owner-occupation can be attributed to the 'Right to Buy' legislation for tenants in social housing (McConaghy *et al.* 2000: 132). In 1998 just under two-fifths of older people who live alone and just under three-quarters who live with a spouse or partner were home owners (see Table 3.1). Most of these older people own their homes outright and this proportion continues to increase as younger generations with higher levels of ownership reach retirement. Table 3.1 also summarizes the type of housing of older people's homes in 1998. Older people living alone are more likely to live in purpose-built flats or maisonettes than other older people are.

In the 1980s elderly people in Britain were more likely than younger people to live in older housing, which was likely to be in poorer condition, lacking in amenities and with sub-standard heating. By 1998 the quality of older people's homes had improved. Only 12 per cent compared with 53 per cent in 1980 were without central heating and only 17 per cent compared with 27 per cent were living in accommodation built before 1918 (Bridgwood 2000: Table 5). However, a survey of housing in England in 1998/99 (McConaghy *et al.* 2000: Table 8G) reported that older householders were more likely to live in relatively low value and smaller accommodation, and were somewhat less likely than other households to have central heating (14 per cent compared with 11 per cent). In both the *General Household Survey* of

Table 3.1   Tenure and type of housing of older people's homes in Britain 1980, 1998

| | Elderly person households | | | | | | Households with no elderly people | |
	Elderly person living alone		Elderly couple		Other elderly households			
	1980 %	1998 %	1980 %	1998 %	1980 %	1998 %	1980 %	1998 %
Tenure:								
Owner-occupied	37	58	54	80	52	76	56	69
Local authority or housing association	47	36	36	16	38	21	33	20
Privately rented	15	6	10	4	9	4	11	11
N=100%	1502	1144	1214	922	744	282	8109	6109
	1980 %	1998 %	1980 %	1998 %	1980 %	1998 %	1980 %	1998 %
Type of housing:								
House or bungalow	64	69	84	89	88	92	82	82
Ground or first-floor flat	30	25	12	8	10	7	13	13
Other flat	6	6	4	3	2	1	5	5
N=100%	1502	1144	1214	922	744	282	8109	6109

Sources: OPCS (1982: Table 10.4) and Bridgwood (2000: Table 6)

1998 (Bridgwood 2000) and the housing survey of 1998/99 (McConaghy *et al.* 2000) older householders were more likely to have under-occupied bedrooms as measured by the 'bedroom standard'.

An important and basic necessity in most northern, central and western European countries is that of adequate heating. Despite the continuing improvements in official indicators of the quality of housing, not least the high proportion of households with central heating, there still remains an annual concern about the impact of hypothermia (Keatinge 1986). The limited data available suggests that older people are still at risk of hypothermia since the presence of central heating does not mean that it is always used owing to low incomes and concerns about being in debt (Hislop *et al.* 1995).

Of course, the objective improvement in older people's housing does not necessarily imply that all older people are experiencing a better quality of life. Official statistics provide a relatively clear picture of some of the objective indicators of the quality of the housing in which people live. But official government surveys fail to routinely assess the physical quality of housing and the way that it is used. This is partly to do with the perceived poor reliability of reported subjective indicators in surveys and partly due to the need for survey designers to maximize the amount of statistical data collected. To get a better picture of the quality of older people's housing we have to rely on ad hoc surveys and small-scale studies that are often challenged as unrepresentative.

Institutional living

Across Europe and throughout history a small proportion of all age groups has lived in an institution of some kind. Contemporary estimates suggest that between 0.5 per cent (Greece) and 9 per cent (the Netherlands) of people aged 65 or over live permanently in long-term care institutions (long-stay hospitals, nursing homes and residential homes) (Pacolet *et al.* 2000: Table 3.4). As mental and physical frailty increases, so older people are increasingly likely to experience institutional living. In Britain at the 1991 Census some 5 per cent of people aged 65 or over, 10 per cent aged 75 or over and 24 per cent aged 85 or over were staying in an institution or communal establishment (OPCS/GRO(S) 1993). So what quality of life do residents experience?

A rich research tradition covering the last five decades has focused on the nature of the institutional environment and the quality of life of older people resident in long-term care institutions. During the 1950s and 1960s the outputs of these studies made depressing reading. Quality of life in older people's homes and long-stay hospitals in the UK was not high. Townsend (1964) highlights the gross inequities between the different kinds of homes in the 1950s.

At one extreme there is the old workhouse with stone floors and unplastered interior walls and long dormitories with ten, twenty and sometimes even fifty iron-framed beds. There are few articles of furniture. Thirty, forty or more persons sit in the huge day rooms, where standards of comfort are minimal. Coarse unpressed clothing with institutional laundry tags is issued. There is no real privacy and little to encourage self-respect...

Clustered in the middle between the extremes are the small buildings converted since the war by local authorities and voluntary associations, usually housing from thirty to fifty persons. In these there are bedrooms for two, three, four and six persons. The bed-frames are usually wooden; many mattresses are interior sprung, and individual or shared wardrobes and dressing tables are provided in addition to chairs and lockers. The rooms are often high and the passages draughty and gloomy; there are ornamental wood carvings and fancy ceilings which are difficult to clean; there are largish gardens or estates and the nearest bus stop and shops are sometimes several hundred yards away at the end of a long drive and a secondary road.

At the other extreme form the old workhouse is the Home built recently as such by the local authority, or the small Home for ten or twenty people run by a voluntary association or a private individual. The quality of such Homes varies widely ... but one of the best examples might be selected. A dozen people live in a fine house overlooking beautiful countryside. They are remote from their relatives and friends and the local community, but they each have their own bed-sitting rooms with fitted carpets, expensive rugs, hand basins, side-tables, not one but two or three wardrobes, chests of drawers, long mirrors, armchairs, pictures, rubber foam mattresses, quilts and three forms of

heating – central heating, electric thermostat fires and electric blankets.
All have their own radios and a few a television set. Some even have a
small electric oven . . .

(Townsend 1964: 223–4)

There was a gradual improvement throughout the last four decades of the
twentieth century in the physical environments of old people's homes and
hospital accommodation. The development of nursing homes in the 1980s as
replacement facilities for long-stay hospitals made little difference to the
general trend. The contrast in physical environments so poignantly described
by Townsend still continues to exist. Some old workhouses continue to be
used as old people's homes or hospitals but they are now few in number and
should be eradicated in the not too distant future. Like the general housing
stock most, probably all, homes are centrally heated but many remain 'cold'
impersonal spaces. New homes tend to be larger and nearly all residents will
have their own small bedroom. The quality of furnishing has improved. The
ubiquitous television and more recently the video recorder have replaced the
radio in the shared living spaces of older people. But as Townsend (1964) and
others have highlighted (Booth 1985; Willcocks *et al.* 1987; Bond *et al.*
1989a), the physical environment is only part of the picture and in con-
sidering the quality of older residents' lives we also need to examine the
social environment of institutional living.

Living in an institution

The social environment of an institution is probably the key to a resident's
quality of life (Challiner *et al.* 1996; Bond 2000). It has long been recognized
(Townsend 1964) that many long-term care institutions, whatever their
clientele, exhibit the characteristics of what Goffman (1961) has termed the
total institution. The characterizing feature of the total institution, which
distinguishes it from other forms of organization, is that unlike life outside
there is no separation between the three central spheres of life: work, leisure
and the family. All aspects of life are conducted within the boundaries of the
institution and under the control of a single authority. Each phase of daily
activities is shared with a large number of other people, all whom are treated
alike and are required to do the same things together. Activities normally
follow a strict routine imposed from above by a system of explicit formal
rulings and a body of officials. The routine of daily activities comprises a
single rational plan that has been designed to fulfil the official aims of the
institution.

Detailed British studies following after Townsend's seminal work (Townsend 1964) continue to find features of the total institution (Booth 1985;
Hughes and Wilkin 1987; Wilkin and Hughes 1987; Willcocks *et al.* 1987;
Bond and Bond 1990; Booth *et al.* 1990). Booth (1985) showed that communal living induces dependency in residents which becomes more severe as
the institutional environment becomes more total. Hughes and Wilkin
(1987) describe how the way physical care is performed reflects and reinforces the 'total' nature of the institution. Willcocks *et al.* (1987) examine the

way that older people's private lives are played out in the public places of residential homes. 'While we can distinguish variation on the basis of staff accounts, we are still left with an overall impression, supported by our observations, that residential life, whatever the setting, is predominantly public and communal, routinised and impersonal' (Willcocks *et al.* 1987: 121). In comparing long-stay hospitals and NHS nursing homes Bond *et al.* (1989b) observed substantial variation in the institutional environments of hospital wards and NHS nursing homes which was associated with quality of life outcomes as measured by the Life Satisfaction Index (Neugarten *et al.* 1961). Although examples of the total institution undoubtedly still exist, and some of the characteristics will always be present, the last forty years has seen continuing development in the quality of institutional environments in response to relentless criticism of the quality of older residents' lives. In Britain, successive governments have been concerned with institutional environments and a number of formal reports have been produced to define clearly the characteristics of the environments which need to be addressed by those responsible for the institutional care of older people (DHSS 1983b; Centre for Policy on Ageing 1984; Wagner 1988). These highlight the importance of autonomy, choice, privacy, social engagement and social participation in the everyday life of older people in institutions. It is therefore not surprising that the way quality of life has been traditionally defined in gerontological research fits so closely the model outlined in Chapter 1.

Living in the community

Returning to the experience of older people living in the community, we observe that social change accelerated during the twentieth century and the world older people were born into was very different to the one in which they are now living out their final years. The impact of two world wars and the rise and fall of communism in Europe, changes in the nature of work and leisure, increasing diversity of cultures, changes in the role of women, family life and social participation makes life at the beginning of the twenty-first century very different to that experienced at the beginning of the twentieth century.

Family and social networks

Changes in the structure of the family and social network reflect changes in population structure. A key development in the twentieth century was the success of modernity in sustaining life and increasing life expectancy. But this has been a different experience for men and women. Women survive longer than men, but as we see later in this chapter those men who do survive have a better health experience than women of the same age. Life expectancy for men aged 65 in 2001 is 81 years and for women 84 years. Consequently the gender (sex) ratio of people aged 65–74 is 123 (i.e. for every 100 men there are 123 women) rising to 289 for people aged 85 or over (ONS 2003). The 2001 projection is that these expectations will increase by a further two years by 2021. This feminization of later life has consequences for the marital status and living arrangements of older people. Due to increased longevity, and the tendency for men to marry women younger than themselves, women are more likely to experience widowhood. Fewer women than men remarry following widowhood or divorce and consequently more older women than older men live alone. The impact of changes in demographic and other social factors such as increased geographical mobility and increasing personal resources in the last five decades is shown in Table 3.2. The notable trend is the decline in the proportion of older people living with others. Data from the 1998 *General Household Survey* show that over half of older people live with a spouse only. Because of widowhood older people aged 85 or over (men: 43 per cent; women: 72 per cent) are more likely to live alone than men and women aged 65–84 (Table 3.3).

Table 3.2 Household structure of elderly people in Britain, 1945–98

	1945* %	1962 %	1976 %	1980 %	1991 %	1998 %
Living alone	10	22	30	34	38	37
Living with spouse only	30	33	44	45	46	51
Living with others	60	44	27	22	15	12

*These data are not nationally representative. See Dale *et al.* (1987) for details.

Sources: Dale *et al.* (1987: Table 1); Goddard and Savage (1994: Table 3); Bridgwood (2000: Table 3)

Table 3.3 Household structure of older people by age, Britain 1998

	65–9 %	70–4 %	75–9 %	80–4 %	85 and over %	All aged 65 and over %
Lone older woman	16	21	34	39	47	26
Lone older man	9	10	11	13	15	10
Living with spouse only	61	57	44	41	25	51
Living with others of same generation	9	7	5	3	4	7
Living with others of younger generation	5	5	6	4	9	6
Total	100	100	100	100	100	100
Base number	*944*	*845*	*699*	*352*	*242*	*3082*

Source: Bridgwood (2000: Table 3)

As we saw in Chapter 2, fifty years ago the extended family was idealized by the community studies in the East End of London (Townsend 1957; Young and Willmott 1957). But it was also recognized that the quality of older people's lives was far from perfect. At the beginning of the twentieth century the structure of family networks had changed with the institutionalization of serial monogamy and a smaller number of family relationships reflecting changes in fertility and family formation. The importance of friends within social networks, particularly for women (Jerrome 1984, 1993; Jerrome and Wenger 1999), is an increasing part of later life. Most older people nowadays, however, are still connected to family-based networks (Phillipson *et al.* 2001). Modern family networks continue to provide emotional, instrumental and financial aid to older people and receive support in return. Interdependency within contemporary networks is no less strong than it was in the past, despite the low prevalence of co-residence and the increasing spatial separation of family networks, not simply across towns and cities but across countries and continents.

Social support

The term social support networks was coined by Wenger (1984) to describe both the structure and the support functions of older people's kin and friendship networks. There is considerable evidence that family and friends provide support to older people especially during times of illness and incapacity. Well-integrated families are assumed to improve the quality of life of family members. But this may not be the case in all families and such cohesion often reflects family and wider cultural expectations than individual preferences. In contrast, individuals who interact infrequently with their older relatives may well begin regular contact at times of crisis and often become long-term informal carers as their elderly relative's health deteriorates. Although the idea of fixed obligations in family life have been challenged by Finch and Mason (1993), there exists empirical support for the idea of a normative hierarchy of informal caregivers (Qureshi and Walker 1989; RIS MRC CFAS 1999). However, as Wenger (1984, 1992) has clearly shown, not everyone is endowed with a social support network capable of maintaining an older person in the community in the face of high physical or psychological dependency. Different types of social network will reflect the availability of close kin, the proportions of family, friends and neighbours involved and the level of interaction that the older person has with members of the network. Different types of network have different potential to provide social support. They may provide a high level of help or very little. This variation in social support networks has an important influence on the quality of life of older people in the community, particularly at times of poor health and illness.

Social participation

The idea of social participation overlaps with social networks. Active participation both formally and informally in the community, whether as regular customers in the local public house or as formal members of churches, clubs and societies, involves others in the older person's social network. Surprisingly little data exists about the daily activities of older people and their social participation. Most surveys have collected information on the contact older people have with relatives, friends and neighbours. About three-quarters of people aged 65 or over see a relative or friend at least once a week and over 80 per cent talk to a neighbour at least once a week (Bridgwood 2000: Tables

40, 42). Contact rates decline with age and the inevitable reduction in social networks as older people's peers die. Data from the Berlin Ageing Study provide insights into the detailed social activity of older people. On an average day (based on the previous day's activities) 45 per cent talked to another person, 17 per cent visited someone, 23 per cent used the telephone, 7 per cent were engaged in church or political activities, 6 per cent helped family members and 2.5 per cent helped other people (Horgas *et al.* 1998: Table 2). However, instrumental activities of daily living such as housework (180 minutes per day) and leisure activities undertaken alone such as reading (93 minutes) and watching TV (163 minutes) account for a large proportion of daily activities. Reported activity levels declined with age.

Standards of living of older people

Although the quality of our lives is not simply about standards of living, for most of us material resources are an important contribution to our life quality. Without an adequate income we would be unable to engage in the variety of activities available to us in the postmodern world. For some, resources may be relatively unimportant, since they seek and enjoy life through spiritual or other means. But for the majority a basic income is essential. An important issue here is what constitutes a basic income to allow a good life?

It has been recognized for some thirty years that what constitutes a basic income is relative. The concept of poverty so clearly delineated by Townsend (1970, 1979) in the 1970s still remains contested, not because of the nature of the concept but in terms of what is essentially an arbitrary political decision. Ever since the emergence of public welfare in Europe different countries have set minimum income levels for different groups within societies. The absolute levels varied between different countries depending on macroeconomic circumstances and ideological positions. In the European Union the minimum basic income or poverty line was set at 50 per cent of average earnings although few member states provide universal support to older citizens at this level (Eurostat 1996: 213). In the UK the poverty line is set lower and has been redefined by successive governments. By 2010 it is estimated that the basic state pension in Britain will be worth less than 25 per cent of average earnings (Atkinson 1995).

In 1978 the Royal Commission on the Distribution of Income and Wealth in the UK reported that one in three older families had incomes on or below the 'poverty line' and that nearly three in every four older families lived on the margins of poverty (Walker 1993). With the rise in owner-occupancy, increases in state pensions during the 1970s and the more general introduction of occupational pension schemes, there is a general belief that current cohorts of older people are better off than earlier generations of older people and families with children. For a minority, who are likely to be younger, male and have been continuously employed in non-manual occupations, there is evidence that this is indeed the case (Falkingham and Victor 1991). For the majority, however, later life is a time of lowering standards of living (Johnson and Falkingham 1992; Walker 1993; Dilnot *et al.*

1994). Income levels have been persistently lower than the general population for a number of decades and the myth of well-off older people arose
because of the relative increase in the number of non-pensioner families in
poverty during the 1980s (Walker 1993). The decline in the basic state
pension since 1984 relative to average earnings continues to have a significant impact on pensioner incomes. The impact on the incomes of older
women has been particularly marked. All pensioners who rely on state
support only (the majority of women) will continue to see a decline in
income and their standard of living as they age.

Routinely published statistics from the Family Resources Survey provide
information about the current incomes of older person households (Semmence *et al.* 2000: Table 3.4). Older person households have much lower
incomes than non-pensioner households. Households with one or more
adults of pensionable age have an average weekly income of £290 compared
with £560 for all households with children.

The incomes of older people are not evenly distributed. Older people in the
top quintile of the income distribution had four times the median income of
older people in the bottom quintile of the income distribution. Inequalities
between rich and poor continue to increase (Dilnot *et al.* 1994), because the
relative value of the basic state pension continues to decline and the savings
and investments of the better-off have provided returns above inflation for
the last thirty years.

Sources of income

There are four major sources of income available to older people: income
from the state, occupational pensions, earnings, and income from savings and
investments. The state has a major direct role in providing incomes for older
people in the UK and other member states of the European Union (Pacolet *et
al.* 2000). In contrast, a higher proportion of younger adults receive income
from earnings. Non-participation in the labour force is the key to inequalities
between older people living on a pension and younger adults and also
accounts for income inequalities among older people (particularly between
men and women). Those older people who are still economically active are
far less likely to be in poverty than those who are inactive. But the proportion
of earned income has declined for many years and continues to decline
(Phillipson 1998). The relative effect of different sources of income for older
people in different quintiles of the income distribution is shown in Table 3.4.
The important sources of income for the top quintile of older people is not
their income from state pensions or other state benefits. Employment
income, occupational pensions, and income from savings and investments
are the key sources of income for this quintile. Previous labour market
experience and particularly the ability to accrue occupational pension contributions as well as the accumulation of savings and investment assets
appear to be the key determinants of high income in later life. Recent fiscal
changes to lower interest rates, the collapse of investment income and
changes to occupational pensions may have differential impact on older
people with savings and investments. However, they will remain relatively

Table 3.4 Pensioners' income by source 1996/97 (incomes per week, 2001/02 prices)

| | Quintiles of the income distribution | | | | | |
	Bottom	2nd	3rd	4th	Top	Overall mean
Pensioner couples	£	£	£	£	£	£
Gross income	152	193	245	342	687	324
Of which:†						
Benefit income	132	151	157	157	134	146
Occupational pension	14	29	60	118	265	97
Investment income	7	9	16	45	166	49
Earnings	*	4	10	21	119	30
Other income	*	1	1	1	3	1
Single pensioners	£	£	£	£	£	£
Gross income	84	115	135	174	321	166
Of which:†						
Benefit income	77	96	110	114	121	104
Occupational pension	3	11	17	36	104	34
Investment income	5	7	7	17	69	21
Earnings	*	*	1	6	23	6
Other income	*	*	*	*	3	1

* Estimates of less than £0.50.
† Columns do not sum to totals because of averaging and rounding.
Source: Davis *et al.* (2003: Table A17)

better off than older people with incomes only from state benefits.

These data mask significant differences between men and women. Retirement policies in the twentieth century, which are based on labour market experience, favoured men. The large majority of women currently receiving pensions will either have been in full-time unpaid employment or will have experienced part-time and disrupted paid employment and lower incomes than men. Women are less likely than men to receive an occupational pension and those who do will find that their income remains substantially lower. In 1997, women aged 65–9 received an average income from occupational pensions of £22 per week compared with £67 per week for men (Phillipson 1998).

Health status in later life

The relationship between quality of life and particularly life satisfaction and health states has been well established (Okun *et al.* 1984; Zautra and Hempel 1984; Kennedy *et al.* 1991). In general poor health is associated with lower life quality. This relationship is probably perceived to be stronger than the epidemiological evidence suggests with the increasing concern of the postmodern individual with health and illness. One of the enduring negative images of later life is that of ill health and disability. Ill health in later life is a source of pain and suffering and can bring many losses to the individual including those of independence and autonomy, self-esteem and dignity, mobility, social interaction and participation in everyday life. But although ill health and disability increase with age, this is not the experience of many during their 'retirement' years.

A number of myths exist about the health of older people, its causes and its consequences (Sidell 1995). A dominant myth about older people in general and about their health specifically is the notion that they are all the same. Although the heterogeneity of older people is now clearly recognized nationally at a policy level (Joint Taskforce on Older People 2000), this has not always been the case. There is now recognition of the substantial evidence to support a picture of a diverse population category not only in terms of age, gender, ethnic and socio-economic background but also in terms of social networks, leisure interests and social participation. A still prevalent myth is one held by many health professionals as well as older people themselves, which Sidell terms as the 'medical myth'. Supported by morbidity statistics is the notion that ageing is synonymous with disease and that any condition that medicine cannot cure is simply 'due to your age'. This is reinforced by health professionals' experience of older people, which is often one of illness and disease. But many older people do not suffer chronic illness and disability and many older people claim good health despite their incapacities.

Increases in life expectancy are one indicator of the improving health status of older people. However, current information suggests that these have not been matched by a proportionate decline in ill health and disability (Medical Research Council 1994). But a further optimistic myth is the view that morbidity will increasingly be compressed into the last few months of the life span. A corresponding idea is the concept of the rectangular survival curve (Fries and Crapo 1981). The argument here is that the present upper limit of 115 years for human longevity is unlikely to be extended in the foreseeable future, but that progress in health and welfare will continue to delay the onset of, and reduce the disabilities associated with, most of the important conditions of later life, thus compressing the bulk of these disorders into a relatively short period, at the far end of life, and so achieve a human survival curve with an approximately rectangular shape. When this model was first proposed some twenty years ago there was little empirical support for its application in European populations. Even though we still await the supporting data, it remains conceptually attractive.

Measuring health status

Population statistics on the health of older people are notoriously difficult to use. Traditionally epidemiologists have used both mortality and morbidity data. Because of the high prevalence of comorbidity in later life both mortality and morbidity statistics may mask what is really going on. By comorbidity is meant the presence of more than one disease or chronic illness; for example many older people will live with arthritis and heart disease. Survey researchers have therefore developed self-report techniques for assessing health status. Yet successive surveys of older people in Europe and North America consistently find that older people rate their health as good while morbidity data suggest that their health is poor. Self-report data may not reflect absolute levels of morbidity, but rather the expectations of older people about their health and the services available to them. However, consistently self-ratings of health have been reliable predictors of survival and mortality (Idler and Benyamini 1997). In gerontological research one response has been to focus on measurement of disability and handicap, although again these often rely on self-report and there are substantial data to suggest that older people's evaluations of their abilities do not necessarily equate with those of other family members or formal health professional assessments. There are complex reasons for such different assessments. We return to these methodological issues in Chapter 6 when discussing the assessment of quality of life in gerontological research. In reviewing published data on health status these caveats should be held strongly in mind. A further caveat about such data is the cultural bias against ethnic minority groups who tend to be under-represented in routine statistics and health surveys relying on self-report (Blakemore and Boneham 1994).

In a British health and lifestyle survey (Blaxter 1990) some 9000 adult respondents were asked about their health and lifestyles, certain aspects of their fitness were measured and they were invited to express their opinions and attitudes towards health and health-related behaviour. Three indices of health were used in the study: a level of fitness based on physiological measures ('fitness/unfitness'); presence of disease and impairment based on reported medically defined conditions and degrees of disability which accompany them ('disease/disability'); and the presence of illness based on reports of symptoms suffered ('illness'). Figure 3.1 shows the marked relationship between chronological age and the three indices used by Blaxter in the British health and lifestyle survey (Blaxter 1990).

Data are collected routinely as part of the annual *General Household Survey* in Britain on reported long-standing illness or limiting long-term illness. Table 3.5 shows changes in the reported prevalence of long-standing illness by age group. Men and women report similar levels of long-standing illness, contradicting other data that suggest that women have higher levels of morbidity than men. Prevalence increases with age for both men and women but reported prevalence declines among people aged 85 or over. Changing expectations about health with age and the high proportion of people aged 85 or over not surveyed because of infirmity or because they are resident in a long-term care institution may explain this anomaly in the data.

Overall these health status measures indicate that a substantial proportion of older people are experiencing ill health and that this increases with age. It is therefore not surprising that health plays such a large part in our thinking and the thinking of older people when reflecting on quality of life.

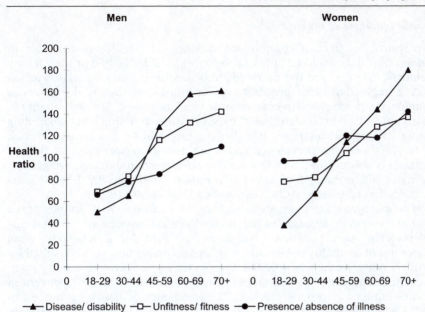

Figure 3.1   Health rates for three dimensions of health by age and gender (total population mean = 100)

Source: Blaxter (1990: Figure 4.1)

Table 3.5   Limiting and non-limiting long-standing illness of men and women in later life by age group, Britain 1998

	65–9	70–4	75–9	80–4	85 or over	All aged 65 or over
Men	%	%	%	%	%	%
Limiting long-standing illness	33	38	41	57	47	40
Non-limiting long-standing illness	26	20	24	14	18	22
No long-standing illness	41	42	35	29	35	38
Base number = 100%	*446*	*386*	*281*	*140*	*83*	*1336*
Women	%	%	%	%	%	%
Limiting long-standing illness	36	41	48	50	54	43
Non-limiting long-standing illness	20	20	16	14	11	18
No long-standing illness	44	39	36	36	35	39
Base number = 100%	*497*	*459*	*418*	*212*	*158*	*1744*
All people aged 65 or over	%	%	%	%	%	%
Limiting long-standing illness	34	40	45	53	51	42
Non-limiting long-standing illness	24	20	20	14	14	19
No long-standing illness	42	40	35	33	35	39
Base number = 100%	*943*	*845*	*699*	*352*	*241*	*3080*

Source: Bridgwood (2000: Table 13)

Physical conditions of later life

Two sources of data of common conditions of later life are available in Britain. Both rely on some kind of self-report by older people or their family members. The first are the morbidity statistics from general practice which usually imply that older people have consulted their family doctor about symptoms which have then been recorded and diagnosed. Some morbidity in general practice will be identified through routine screening and case finding during ad hoc consultations, but the majority will be due to self-referral. Table 3.6 shows the prevalence (rates per 10,000 person years at risk) of common conditions in later life for men and women in different age groups. Estimates are presented of selected common conditions by International Classification of Disease (ICD) chapter headings (WHO 1992).

Of people aged 65 or over, diseases of the circulatory system, diseases of the respiratory system, diseases of the musculoskeletal system and mental disorders were most prevalent. Neoplasms account for a relatively small proportion of morbidity in later life. The highest proportion who consulted for cancer among women was of the breast and of the prostate among men. Endocrine, nutritional and metabolic diseases account for about 5 per cent of all consultations in general practice. The prevalence of diabetes is highest in the 75–84 age group and is more common among men than women. Diseases of the blood are relatively uncommon in general practice. The prevalence of iron deficiency anaemia increases with age and is highest for older women. Mental disorders in later life generate substantial general practice activity. The most common are neurotic disorders with a significantly higher prevalence among women. The prevalence of dementia is lower than epidemiological studies. This probably reflects the relatively low rate of self-referral and the use of different diagnostic criteria. Among older people Parkinson's disease and disorders of the external ear are relatively common diseases of the nervous system with prevalence higher among men than women. Diseases of the circulatory system are common conditions of later life. Hypertensive disease, ischaemic heart disease and cerebrovascular disease all contribute substantially to general practice morbidity among patients aged 65 or over. But the single group of diseases that generates most practice activity among older people is acute respiratory infections. Chronic obstructive pulmonary disease is also a significant contributor to illness in later life. The prevalence of constipation is high among older people, particularly those aged 85 or over as are infections of the urinary tract. The most prevalent chronic condition of later life is osteoarthritis, particularly among women.

The second source of data is the *General Household Survey* that relies solely on the self-reports of respondents living in private households. Long-standing conditions reported by older men and women are shown in Table 3.7. Diseases of the musculoskeletal system were reported by 24 per cent of men and 36 per cent of women aged 65 or over and diseases of the heart and circulatory system by 29 per cent of men and 28 per cent of women. Other conditions were reported by less than one in ten of older people. On average older people with a long-standing illness reported 1.7 conditions (Bridgwood 2000: Table 17), indicating substantial comorbidity.

Table 3.6 Prevalence of common selected conditions of later life, England and Wales 1991–92 (rates per 10,000 person years at risk)*

	Men			Women		
	65–74	75–84	85+	65–74	75–84	85+
Neoplasms						
Cancer of the trachea, bronchus and lung (ICD 162)	45	61	71	15	17	16
Cancer of the breast (ICD 174)	–	–	–	81	88	87
Cancer of the prostate (ICD 185)	45	137	155	–	–	–
Cancer of the bladder (ICD 188)	27	50	71	3	12	18
Endocrine, nutritional and metabolic disease						
Acquired hypothyroidism (ICD 244)	42	48	49	245	204	193
Diabetes mellitus (ICD 250)	428	475	327	337	274	238
Gout (ICD 274)	197	180	178	53	68	73
Obesity (ICD 278)	62	21	–	135	51	12
Diseases of the blood						
Iron deficiency anaemia (ICD 280)	70	121	184	101	212	266
Mental disorders						
Senile dementia (ICD 290)	10	97	309	18	139	307
Neurotic disorders (ICD 300)	257	244	226	582	508	398
Depressive disorder not elsewhere classified (ICD 311)	94	112	190	174	207	175
Diseases of the nervous system and sense organs						
Parkinson's disease (ICD 332)	64	149	155	51	91	128
Disorders of the external ear (ICD 380)	851	1005	927	546	681	727
Diseases of the circulatory system						
Hypertensive disease (ICD 401–405)	1482	1124	505	1773	1606	715
Ischaemic heart disease (ICD 410–414)	920	915	879	498	675	597
Cerebrovascular disease (ICD 430–438)	272	546	749	177	417	723
Varicose veins (ICD 454)	197	232	232	263	307	244
Haemorrhoids (ICD 455)	159	143	125	140	118	91
Diseases of the respiratory system						
Acute respiratory infections (ICD 460–466)	1936	2268	2716	2201	2170	2480
Chronic obstructive pulmonary diseases (ICD 490–496)	886	1032	1105	691	676	534
Diseases of the digestive system						
Constipation (ICD 564)	169	396	683	181	337	554
Diseases of the genitourinary system						
Urinary tract infection (ICD 599)	265	440	636	464	600	831
Diseases of the musculoskeletal system						
Rheumatoid arthritis (ICD 714)	69	52	18	133	122	85
Osteoarthritis (ICD 715)	818	1017	1022	1217	1581	1584
Injury and poisoning						
Fracture of the neck of femur (ICD 820)	5	18	89	23	63	193

*Person years at risk is the sum of the number of days each patient in sex/age group category was registered with a study practice during the year, divided by the number of days in the year.
Source: McCormick *et al.* (1995: Tables: 2I, 2K, 2L, 2N, 2O, 2P, 2Q, 2R, 2T and 2W)

Table 3.7 Reported long-standing conditions in later life of men and women by age group, Britain 1998 (rates per 1000)

Condition group		65–9	70–4	75–9	80–4	85 and over	65 and over
Musculoskeletal system	Men	210	257	203	336	277	240
	Women	329	353	426	354	361	364
Heart and circulatory system	Men	271	273	306	343	265	286
	Women	264	277	289	307	278	280
Respiratory system	Men	94	106	78	179	96	103
	Women	79	89	96	75	63	84
Endocrine and metabolic	Men	87	68	96	57	72	79
	Women	103	124	84	80	82	99
Digestive	Men	67	36	57	43	96	55
	Women	56	76	67	104	82	72
Eye complaints	Men	36	31	57	71	133	49
	Women	24	52	62	94	171	63
Nervous system	Men	38	34	39	14	24	34
	Women	26	39	43	33	44	36
Bases = 100%	*Men*	*447*	*385*	*281*	*140*	*83*	*1336*
	Women	*496*	*459*	*418*	*212*	*158*	*1743*

Source: Bridgwood (2000: Table 18)

Mental health

Physical ill health is often compounded by mental health problems. Dementia, probably one of the most feared conditions of later life, affects about 5 per cent of people aged 65 or over at any one time. Epidemiological evidence shows a doubling of the prevalence of dementia every seven years (Jorm *et al.* 1987), with up to 20 per cent of those aged 80 or over having the condition (MRC CFAS 1998).

More prevalent are depression and other functional psychiatric illnesses for which there exists no identified organic cause. Depression is probably *the* epidemic condition of later life. Prevalence estimates are notoriously unreliable, however, ranging from 6 to 26 per cent in British studies (Brayne and Ames 1988). Psychological well-being would therefore appear to be a considerable component of the quality of later life.

Disability

Gerontological research has a long tradition in assessing disability as a more useful strategy for measuring outcomes of health and interventions and for planning health and social care services for older people. Again a challenge to this approach is the self-report nature of disability and the impact that the different expectations of older people may have. Under-reporting of disability may occur because disability is seen as a natural part of normal ageing. Men and women, people from different generations and socio-economic or ethnic groups will report disability in a variety of ways because of different cultural experiences and expectations.

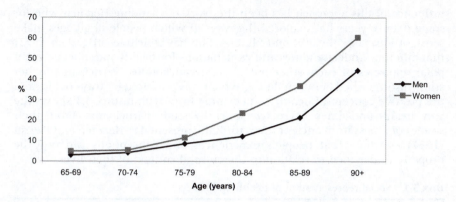

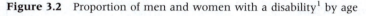

Figure 3.2   Proportion of men and women with a disability[1] by age

[1] Activities of daily living score 11–18

Source: MRC CFAS (Medical Research Council Cognitive Function and Ageing Study) (2001: Table 2)

Like poor health status and morbidity, the prevalence of disability increases with age (Figure 3.2). Recent estimates suggest that in England and Wales some 1.3 million people over the age of 65 are experiencing moderate or severe disability (MRC CFAS and RIS MRC CFAS 1999). Like health status, functional ability is likely to have a marked influence on the way older people think about their quality of life. As we saw in Chapter 1, it has clearly influenced the way gerontologists think about the concept.

Experiencing ill health

There has been a lot of attention in both the sociology of health and illness and health psychology on the experience of illness, disease and disability. Particular foci have been about the impact of illness on everyday life, the meaning it has for the individual and the way people respond to the experience. Although not specifically about later life, a number of the contributions are about older people or about chronic conditions that are more prevalent in later life.

One important aspect is the way that older people perceive or conceptualize health and ill health. In industrialized societies lay concepts of health are likely to include biomedical explanations of health since we have all been taught to think, at least in part, in biomedical terms. The media regularly reinforces these when announcing the latest breakthrough for conditions like heart disease and Alzheimer's disease. Yet although 'educated' lay people may accept and take for granted biological knowledge such as the germ theories of disease, it is clear from a number of studies that lay explanations of health are often complex, subtle and sophisticated and based on other data.

One approach to the study of lay perceptions of health uses the Durkheimian notion of *social representation* (Durkheim 1964). An important influence of this approach has been the work of Claudine Herzlich who for some twenty years has explored the ways in which people of all ages make sense of ideas like 'health' and 'illness'. She has concluded (Herzlich 1973) that different understandings and explanations for health and illness are not polar opposites of each other but discrete conceptions. Participants in her study distinguished between illness, which was produced by ways of life, and the positive concept of health, which came from within. Box 3.1 shows the way health and illness were *represented* by study participants. From their studies of illness from ancient times until the present day Herzlich and Pierret (1987) conclude that people's experiences and conceptions can only be properly understood in relation to the cultural context of their lives.

Box 3.1   Social representation of health and illness

Descriptions of health
Health in a vacuum – absence of disease
Reserve of health – physical robustness and resistance to illness
Equilibrium – positive well-being or internal harmony and balance

Descriptors of illness
Illness as destroyer – inability to continue 'normal' life activities
Illness as liberator – freedom from responsibilities
Illness as occupation – a challenge to overcome and focus in life

---

Source: Herzlich (1973)

Blaxter and Paterson (1982) and Williams (1983) in separate British studies showed that health can be presented by older people in similar ways to Herzlich's respondents. Health was perceived negatively, as the absence of illness, functionally, as the ability to cope with everyday activities, or positively, as fitness or well-being. Since within the modern world health continues to have a moral dimension, ill health and moral wrong-doing are interconnected. Health can therefore be seen in terms of will power, self-discipline and self-control. In the *Health and Lifestyle Survey* Blaxter (1990) reported nine different lay definitions of health (see Box 3.2). Most respondents to the survey offered multiple concepts of health. The kinds of definitions reported, however, varied by gender and life cycle position. Older people, particularly older men, focused on function, although ideas about contentment and happiness were commonplace.

The impact of chronic illness on the lives of older people has been well documented both in social science research and literature. A number of key themes have emerged: disrupted biographies (Bury 1982), the loss of self (Charmaz 1987), the search for meaning (Bury 1988); coping with uncertainty (Pinder 1988) and the impact on significant others (Anderson 1988; Corbin and Strauss 1988).

From his discussions with patients attending a rheumatology outpatient clinic Bury (1982) coined the term biographical disruption to describe the development of a chronic illness and its psychosocial consequences, including quality of life, for the individual concerned. Chronic illness is one of those

Box 3.2   Lay definitions of health

Definition	Sample response
Health:	
As not ill	Someone I know who is very healthy is me, because I haven't been to a doctor yet.
Despite disease	I am very healthy despite this arthritis.
As a reserve	Both parents are still alive at 90 so he belongs to healthy stock.
As 'the healthy life'	I call her healthy because she goes jogging and doesn't eat fried food.
As physical fitness	There's tone to my body, I feel fit.
As energy or vitality	Health is when I feel I can do anything.
As social relationships	You feel as though everyone is your friend. I enjoy life more, and can work, and help other people.
As function	She's 81 and she gets her work done quicker than me, and she does the garden.
As psychosocial well-being	Well I think health is when you feel happy.

Source: Blaxter (1990: Chapter 2)

life experiences in which the normal structures of everyday life and the forms of knowledge that underpin them are disrupted. But chronic illness does not mean just the disruption to our taken-for-granted assumptions and behaviour about our everyday lives or the experience of suffering in terms of pain and changes to our social lives. Chronic illness also triggers self-reflection and the need to rethink one's own biography and concept of self.

In order to define strategies adopted by individuals in their management of chronic illness we need to understand *their* meaning of chronic illness. In doing this Bury (1988) distinguishes meaning as consequence and meaning as significance. Consequences of chronic illness are often articulated in practical and policy terms. Chronic illness can lead to disability and loss of function and to handicap. It is an experience that is characterized as a problem for individuals because of loss of social function and the costs that such loss entails. It leads to increasingly restrictive lives, social isolation and loneliness. Equally it has a marked impact on significant others whose life patterns can be dramatically challenged by the emergence of chronic illness (Anderson 1988; Corbin and Strauss 1988).

At the same time chronic illness is problematized by society. The second level of meaning is its significance characterized by stigmatization, marginalization of the individual, being discredited by others, and the perceived burden on others. For (Charmaz 1983), therefore, chronic illness results in a fundamental loss of self as individuals see their former self-images crumbling away. The process of adaptation may reflect individuals' attempts to redefine self and engage coping strategies, which inevitably involve redefining their own quality of life. A key challenge in this process is that of uncertainty and the complexity of the issues that have to be worked through by the person with chronic illness and their significant others.

Experiencing quality of life

In this chapter we have taken a fairly traditional approach focusing on the social contexts of people's lives. This has led us to examine and reflect on some of the constituent elements of life quality identified in the model presented in Chapter 1. In particular we have focused on social and material resources – the physical and social environments in which older people live, their standard of living and, because of its dominance in the minds of many older people, the experience of health and illness in later life. Much of this chapter has provided social epidemiological evidence. But although there undoubtedly exists in statistical terms at least an association between good life quality and access to social and material resources this may not be the best way to examine quality of life. There still exists the conundrum emerging from a variety of studies suggesting that some people who are disadvantaged, whether it be in terms of their standard of living or physical environment, their social resources or their health status, report, and appear to have, a good quality of life. To answer this we need to examine the relationship between the self and society and reflect on what this relationship means to our understanding of quality of life. But to do this we need to think more broadly and reconsider the role of the self in society and try to bridge the gaps between society and the individual and structure and agency in our social gerontological theory. Equally we need to examine some of the methods used to capture the quality of older people's lives in gerontological studies and re-examine them within the context of the relationship between the individual and society. The next three chapters attempt to achieve these tasks.

4

Quality of life and the postmodern world

People see you and think 'old'. And they think they should treat you differently, just because they've decided that you're 'old'. So they shout at you, they do, they raise their voices as if you're deaf, and they shout, and everyone can hear what they're saying. But then, I calmly say to them would you like me to speak to you as if you were a child? No, so don't speak to me as if I am, thank you very much...

(Corner 1999: 239 [1;13;1[1]])

How other people see us, how they relate to us, how they speak to us and how they treat us influences the way we perceive our quality of life. A key process is the way others typify (Schutz 1972) individuals when they meet them, a process summed up so cogently by the quote from the participant in Corner's study: 'People see you and think "old".' We all use typifications in everyday life as part of making sense of daily life and our interaction with others. Often our typifications may appear inappropriate to the subject of our typification as illustrated by the above quotation. This is because many typifications we use are based on stereotypes, many of which are negative. In this chapter we explore many of the stereotypes of older people and seek to understand the way these are presented in the public sphere – in public life, the media and the world of art and literature. We will try to understand images of ageing as presented in our twenty-first-century world. To do this we will draw on the work of a number of authors but particularly Blaikie, Featherstone and Hepworth (Featherstone and Hepworth 1989, 1993; Featherstone and Wernick 1995; Blaikie and Hepworth 1997; Blaikie 1999; Hepworth 2000). By investigating public images of ageing we hope to provide some insight into the relationship between the images and stereotypes of ageing and the experiences of older people and their quality of life. In order to do this we need to explore the cultural representations of traditional and modern images of ageing. We will then consider the evidence of ageing stereotypes. Finally we will examine the way that our stereotypes and images affect the inner worlds of older people and how they influence and reproduce ageism.

Representations of later life

Images of ageing may use oral and written language as well as other medians such as photographs and film. All images provide a symbolic representation of reality. Images of the ageing body that readily come to mind when we think of older people such as wrinkles and grey hair are ones which are readily represented in the public arena, in the media, popular and traditional culture. Such representations are normally self-evident, because of their tangible and mimetic qualities. But we should not be misled by the self-evident and common-sense nature of such images. They are only representatives of a particular symbolic order defined within a specific culture or society.

> Visual images are not simply just direct copies, made with varying degrees of skill and accuracy, from an independently observed external reality, but are, as the word 'image' suggests, the combined product of technical skill and human imagination.
>
> (Blaikie and Hepworth 1997: 102)

Thus wrote Blaikie and Hepworth (1997) in their introduction to a comparative analysis of representations of old age in Victorian painting and contemporary photography. The key idea here is human imagination, of course not withstanding the necessity of artistic skill. Since human imagination will be influenced by culturally determined ideas and practices, images of older people provided within the visual arts are produced within the context of time and place, and reflect the meaning of old age within a particular culture.

A good example is the way in which different cultures interpret the images of contrasting body shapes. Beauty is in the eye of the beholder. It is not a given or necessarily a fixed image of beauty but just a specific symbolic representation within the context of a given culture. Another example is that of the interpretation of the facial wrinkle on older women in different cultures. In China, her grandchildren greet the wrinkle on the Chinese grandmother with joy because it is a sign of high status. In contrast the wrinkle is treated as a sign of bodily and moral decay in many western cultures (Featherstone and Hepworth 1993: 306).

In contemporary American films Markson and Taylor (2000) found gender differences in the way older people were portrayed. Men were more likely to be depicted as vigorous, employed and involved in same-gender friendships and adventure. Older women, in contrast, remained either peripheral to the action or were portrayed as rich dowagers, wives, mothers or lonely spinsters. Older people are rarely represented in advertisements, even when products are being marketed for older consumers. When older people are used as models in advertisements, they tend to be depicted in ways that suggest negative stereotypes of old age (Carrigan and Szmigin 2000).

Images and the human body

The human body has always been a central focus of the biomedical sciences, but social theory neglected the importance of the human body for the understanding of human relations until relatively recently. It is only within the last twenty-five years that this neglect has been addressed, with an outpouring of academic writings about the social body. Nettleton (1995) reflects on the cultural, political and social drivers of this development. First there has been a determined effort by women to reclaim control over their own bodies from a male-dominated medical profession. Feminists have highlighted the way men continue to exploit women through their representation of the physical body. Second, biomedical technological innovation associated with human reproduction has emphasized the confusion in distinguishing the boundary between the physical and social body. Third, ethical debates about the status of human embryos, the actual beginning and ending of human life and who should have control over the use of human bodies for biomedical research, have fuelled academic interest in the social body. Fourth, the development of the consumer society and the increasing commercial interest in keeping the body fit, slim and young (Featherstone 1991) has increased the fascination of postmodernists over the body. Finally, the greying of the population has highlighted the nature of the ageing social body and fuelled debates on euthanasia as well as providing increased opportunities for the commodification of ageing individuals' fears and desires (Gilleard and Higgs 2000).

Irrespective of the development of a sociology of the body, there exists in the public's perception the given that ageing is a bodily affair. This is partly determined by society's preoccupation with health, illness and mortality underpinned by our common-sense knowledge of the body, the biomedical focus on the biological body and the biomedicalization of ageing. Even Gilleard and Higgs (2000) in their polemic *Cultures of Ageing* begrudgingly accept the centrality of the ageing body:

> Faced with the physicality of old age – the changes in appearance and function that are seen socially as defining adult ageing – it seems impossible to argue that ageing can be understood as rooted not in the domain of biology but in social relations. It is in the biological materiality of the body that the 'cultural' approach toward understanding ageing meets its greatest challenge.
>
> (Gilleard and Higgs 2000: 130)

Traditional and modern images

Featherstone and Hepworth (1993) in their influential overview of the images of ageing distinguish between traditional and modern images of ageing as well as emphasizing the continuities between them. Gerontologists now routinely debunk the myth of the 'good old days', in which it was believed that older people lived in a more age-reverent society. The physical appearance of age has never been venerated. Wealth and power were the main source of reverence in earlier times (Laslett 1977) and they probably remain the same in our postmodern world. Perhaps the most noteworthy feature of traditional images of ageing recorded by historians remains one of frailty and dependency, an image still portrayed today. Drawing on the analysis by Tamke (1978) of children's stories, songs and games in nine-teenth-century England, Featherstone and Hepworth (1993) emphasize the threefold distinction between the 'good old', the 'bad old' and those who are simply 'past it'. The good old are 'wise and moral old people who are essentially passive; when they function actively they do so largely through or for other people, primarily children. They teach wisdom and good behaviour to children or, if they are wealthy, they can function as gift-givers.' The bad old are 'foolish and malevolent old people whose conduct is inappropriate to their role as envisaged in Victorian society. They disregard, often flaunt, social conventions by remaining active and self-directed.' The simply past it are 'old people who exhibit no behaviour and, therefore, are neither good nor bad but simply old' (Tamke 1978: 64). Featherstone and Hepworth suggest that these images have roots deep in history, but note that they are also subject to change and may be moulded and reconstructed in attempting to change attitudes towards older people in contemporary society.

Within modern times three key factors would appear to have been influential in changing the perceptions of traditional images over time. First, changes in our perceptions of ageing reflect the increasing celebration of youth culture and the energy and vigour of youth, and the ability of young people to adjust to a rapidly changing world. Accelerating technological change renders the skills and knowledge of older generations redundant; older people are consequently devalued and seen as inappropriate for many roles in modern industrial production. Shortages of skilled young people in the future, of course, may reverse this trend.

Second, there has been increasing age consciousness reflected in the pre-occupation of the media to give the age of perpetrators of crimes, even relatively trivial civil misdemeanours such as parking and speeding offences. Age-consciousness is a product of modernization (Featherstone and Hepworth 1993) and the emergence of an age-stratified society (Riley *et al.* 1972). Experts such as medical scientists, psychologists, management consultants, social administrators and others have developed traditional age categories. This professional or expert knowledge has infiltrated lay knowledge and altered the nature of traditional images of ageing.

The third factor has been the establishment of a global consumer culture, itself a product of modernization. This has contributed to a commodification of ageing, where commodification is the process of taking a good or service that has been produced and used and turning it into an item that is exchanged for money (Estes *et al.* 2001). The production of ageing 'cures' and skin treatments are examples of commodification. Older people are now increasingly seen as a major new market segment based on the emergence of third agers with incomes and assets available for use within an active consumer retirement (Sawchuk 1995).

Stereotypes of older people

A classic stereotype of old age is that of the image of the ageing body portrayed in contrast to the ideal fit body of youth. Youthful bodies are represented as having beauty, energy, grace, moral fortitude and optimism. Ageing bodies represent ugliness, idleness, degeneration and moral failure. These are, of course, stereotypes and we could all provide examples of ugly younger people and beautiful older people even within the limits of our culture. These symbolic polarities, like the use of the black and white contrast in everyday language, are not fixed and will change with changes in context. But stereotypes of older people go beyond the simple images of the ageing body. They incorporate moral interpretations of the physical decline of the 'normal ageing' body to describe behavioural and attitudinal aspects. Robert Butler in his formulation of ageism suggests that older people are perceived as senile, rigid in thought and manner, and old-fashioned in morality and skills (Butler 1987). Most of these stereotypes are negative. Another aspect of stereotypes is their generalization. The process of generalization is common in everyday life. It is a process we generally adopt in making sense of people's actions and behaviours. But it is also a process we use in 'scientific' research (Johnson and Bytheway 1993). 'As people age they are increasingly likely to experience memory problems and be at risk of dementia' is often the conclusion reached in gerontological research. But the fact that the majority of older people never have dementia is ignored and the scientific conclusion reinforces the negative stereotype of senility described by Butler. Negative stereotypes are of course an important aspect of ageism, a concept that we return to below.

An important aspect of the negative stereotyping of older people is the stigmatizing effect on everyday interactions and the quality of life experienced by older people. Our negative stereotypes of older people reflect each of three types of stigma first delineated by Goffman (1968). Images of physical impairments: wrinkles, baldness, stooping and limping are stigmatized characteristics of individuals. 'Blemishes of individual character' such as being rigid in thought and old-fashioned are inferred of older people. Even the 'tribal' behaviour of different generations produces stigmatized effects. A ubiquitous feature of the stigmatizing of individuals is the development of a negative discourse. We use specific words in everyday life such as 'wrinkly', 'crumbly', 'grouchy', 'gaga', 'senile' and 'biddy' as metaphors, without giving thought to their original meaning. And we tend to impute a wide range of imperfections on the basis of the original meaning of the word, a process which reinforces negative stereotypes. Noticeably such terms are not only used by younger people; older people also hold strong stereotypes of others of the same age or generation (Giles and Coupland 1991). Attempts to introduce 'political correctness' in our everyday language will probably fail until our underlying images and stereotypes of later life change.

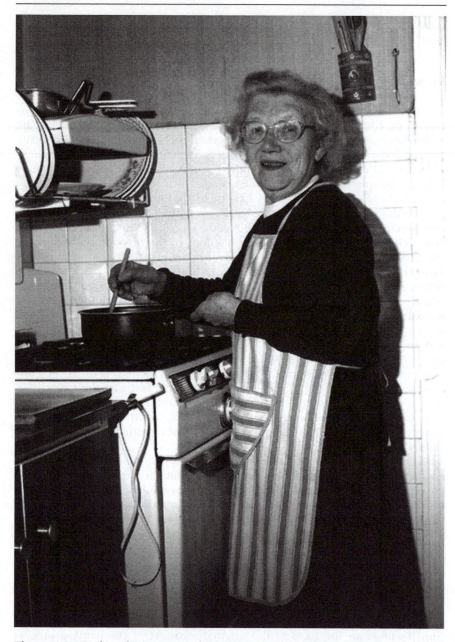

Figure 4.1   Cooking for one at aged 84 (courtesy of Dan Bolam)

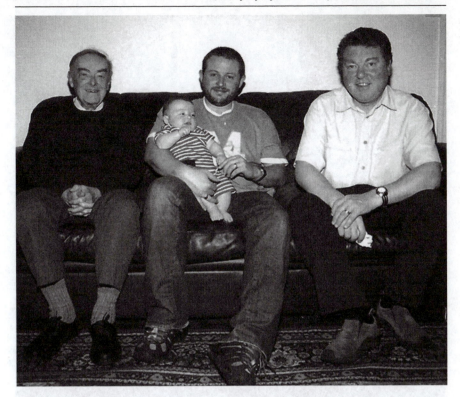

Figure 4.2 Four generations of males (courtesy of Dan Bolam)

The mask of ageing

That older people use the same stigmatizing language to describe others does not necessarily imply that they see themselves as they see others. Comfort (1977) quotes Proust's description of his return to a house he knew and the difficulty he had in recognizing people he knew in his youth:

> A name was mentioned to me, and I was dumbfounded at the thought that it applied to the blonde waltzing girl I had once known and to the stout white-haired lady now walking in front of me. We did not see our own appearance, our own age, but each, like a facing mirror, saw the other's.
>
> (Comfort 1977: 20–1)

Neither Proust nor his former dancing partner may feel old. For some 'old people are in fact young people inhabiting old bodies' (Comfort 1977: 21). For Comfort, ageing is about personal attitude:

> Ageing has no effect upon you as a person. When you are 'old' you feel no different and be no different from what you are now or were when you were young, except that more experiences will have happened. In

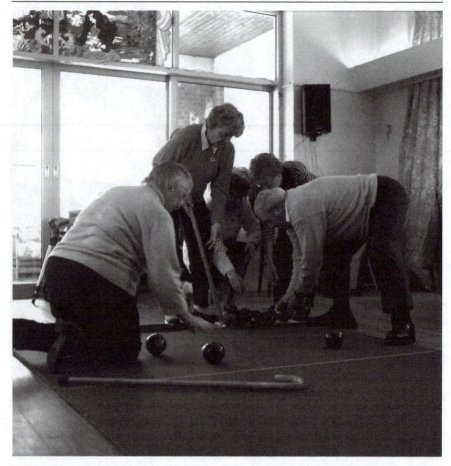

Figure 4.3   Communal fun in a sheltered housing complex (courtesy of Dan Bolam)

age your appearance will change, however, you may encounter more physical problems. When you do, these will affect you only as physical problems affect a person of any age. An 'aged' person is simply a person who has been there longer than a young person.

(Comfort 1977: 28)

Such an attitude has been immortalized in a book title, *I Don't Feel Old*, and the prescient quotation with which we headed Chapter 2:

It doesn't matter how old you are, it's how you feel, isn't it?

(Thompson *et al.* 1991: 107)

It is also a sentiment reported by the distinguished author J. B. Priestley when he was asked on the occasion of the publication of his ninety-ninth work what it was like being old:

It is as though walking down Shaftesbury Avenue as a fairly young man, I was suddenly kidnapped, rushed into a theatre and made to don the grey hair, the wrinkles and other attributes of age, then wheeled on stage. Behind the appearance of age I am the same person, with the same thoughts, as when I was younger.

(Puner 1974: 7)

Such attitudes or opinions encouraged Featherstone and Hepworth to refer to the mask of ageing (Featherstone and Hepworth 1989, 1991, 1995), in which the ageing body masks the inner and youthful self unable to represent the inner self adequately. For the ageing individual 'continuity is maintained by a youthful or timeless identity, while discontinuity is experienced through the progressive betrayals of the body' (Biggs 1999: 67–8). This version of the use of the metaphor has been rejected as a postmodernist denial of ageing (Andrews 1999). But from the perspective of analytical psychology the metaphor describes the mask as one rooted in social conformity. Biggs explains:

Continuity is more easily held by the body as the physical centre of personal experience, while the self is marked by transcendent change . . . it is the self that experiences the discontinuity of the first and second halves of life and expands as a result of new challenges and new psychological contents becoming available to consciousness.

(Biggs 1999: 69)

In other words there exists a disparity between the public images of ageing and the private or personal internal experiences of ageing. This contrast gives prominence to the idea that old age is a mask, which conceals the real self.

But our images of ageing remain dominated by physical appearance and the way others interact with us. Changes in physical appearance have been credited by feminists (Macdonald and Rich 1984) with the increasing invisibility of older women in society. The experience of everyday life suggests that older women are stigmatized by physical appearance. In interactions with others it is the younger woman to whom others turn. For example, Rich found that when she accompanied Macdonald, an older woman, into a shop, it was the younger woman to whom the shop assistant responded despite being addressed by the older woman. In the cited example the shop assistant was male and, depending on relative age, sexual attractiveness may have played some role here. However, in other circumstances shop assistants who are female and older may display the same behaviour, illustrating yet again the insidious nature of ageism.

Ageism

A previous book in the *Rethinking Ageing* series has comprehensively addressed ageism and associated age prejudice (Bytheway 1995). Bytheway reviewed contemporary discourses on ageism and described a range of settings in which ageism is clearly influencing the quality of life of older people. It is not our intention to repeat this eloquent contribution to our

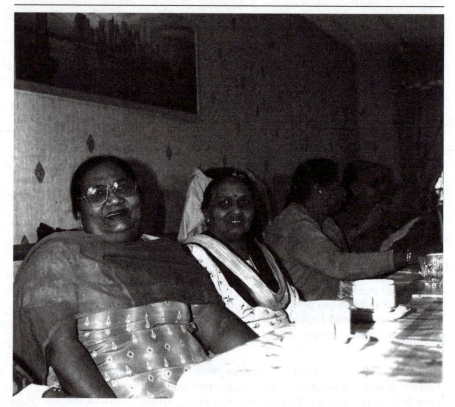

Figure 4.4 Older Asian women enjoying a meal (courtesy of Dan Bolam)

understanding of quality of life. But it would be remiss of us if we did not revisit some of the issues highlighted, since ageism is such an important characteristic of twenty-first-century life.

Ageism, the negative stereotyping of individuals on the basis of age, is institutionalized in the UK and other European societies. Ageism has long been recognized as contributing to the quality of life of older people. Butler (1987) made the direct link between the two other processes whereby the injustice of discrimination is experienced by individuals exhibiting distinct biological characteristics, namely racism and sexism. His well-known definition is widely quoted:

> Ageism is defined as a process of systematic stereotyping of, and discrimination against, people because they are old, just as racism and sexism accomplish this for skin colour and gender.
>
> (Butler 1987: 22)

In a book concerned with older people, and by reproducing Butler's definition, it would be easy to promulgate the myth that ageism is solely about older people. But of course ageism, like ageing, affects people of all ages (Itzin 1986). 'It is a prejudice based on age not old age' (Johnson and Bytheway

1993). But we strongly associate ageism with old age. Many biological theories of ageing and the traditional stereotypes of later life discussed above highlight the association of ageing with biological decline. This reinforces the use of ageism to describe the oppression of older people. For the remainder of our discussion we refer to ageism in later life and reflect on the impact of ageism on the quality of life of older people.

The institutionalization of ageism in later life is reinforced by the legal, political, educational, and health and welfare structures of modern society. Ageism is also internalized in the attitudes of individuals towards older people, which are reinforced by these same structures in society. Employment law and practice, for example, now provide for equal opportunities for women and oppressed minorities and outlaw job discrimination on the basis of gender, race, sexual orientation and disability. But age has been excluded from this legislation. Consequently older people continue to be discriminated against on the basis of age in the job market (Laczko and Phillipson 1990, 1991; Walker and Taylor 1993). Age discrimination against older people in health and welfare services was unrecognized for many years (Henwood 1990). But the rationing of medical treatments and health services on the basis of increasing age continues (Bond 1997). It remains to be seen whether policy changes that recognize age discrimination and ageism in health care eradicate these processes in the delivery of health and social care in the future (DoH 2001).

We have seen how people's attitudes towards older people are influenced by images of ageing. One way in which ageism is conceptually different from racism and sexism is the fact that if we all live long enough, an increasingly high probability, we will be old enough to experience ageism in later life. For white men experience of discrimination on the basis of gender or skin colour is unlikely. Comfort (1977) forcibly illustrates the potential impact of this distinction for older people in the future:

> Unless we are old already, then the next 'old people' will be us. Whether we go along with the kind of treatment meted out to those who are now old depends upon how fast society can sell us the kind of pup it sold them and it depends more upon that than upon any research. No pill or regimen known or likely could transform the latter years of life as fully as could a change in our vision of age and a militancy in attaining that change.
>
> (Comfort 1977: 13)

Ageist attitudes reinforce age discrimination in the public services. Clinical decisions about medical treatments are likely to be made on the basis of attitudes about normal ageing, a concept we turn to below but summed up in the often heard comment: 'What do you expect at your age?' Ageist attitudes are widely reported in long-term care. Health and social care workers have been observed to express ageist attitudes by invoking cultural metaphors of childhood and labelling patients and residents as 'in their second childhood' (Hazan 1980; Bond 1993a; Hockey and James 1993; Becker 1994). Such professional practices may be seen as an unfortunate but inevitable response to human dependency. But the use of metaphoric strategies of infantilization is just one means of creating and maintaining the powerful social divisions between them, the 'aged' and 'infirm', and us, the younger and abler members of society.

Older people's responses to ageism

The oppressive and institutionalized nature of ageism inevitably means that we are all ageist much of the time and older people are ageist against themselves. Corner (1999) in her study of the public and private accounts (Cornwell 1984) of older people, found that ageism was a significant theme that emerged from participants' public accounts. The language of older participants (average age 77) was principally negative. It reflected that used by the media when describing old age, longevity and the increasing numbers of older people. Participants talked of the problems of old age and the burden of the ageing population. They were concerned about becoming a burden themselves. They conformed to ageist stereotypes. The participants' stereotype of older people was one of a homogeneous group, synonymous with ill health, even if this had not been their own personal experience. Corner also found that participants presented passive attitudes and appeared to conform to ageist stereotypes of 'the nice old lady' (participants were predominantly female).

One aspect of ageism, which is well documented and which we have already alluded to, is the rationing of health services on the basis of age (Henwood 1990). In Corner's study many were aware of the health services' need to ration and prioritize services and the demand for other public service resources associated with population growth and the ageing of the population, such as pensions and social security benefits. Participants also introduced the concept of need and the prioritizing of resources for 'those who needed them most' (Corner 1999: 215). For Corner's older participants those most in need were children and younger adults, those who have 'the chance of a whole life ahead of them'. In their public accounts they treated it as a moral issue and one where certain social groups were more deserving of care than older people were, although male participants stressed ideas of entitlement. Thus the almost unanimous acceptance of the devalued position of older people in society militated against challenging or even questioning ageism in society.

How do the ageist attitudes of older people influence their quality of life? Corner's study provides insight into the way ageism impacts on older people through the interpretation of private accounts of study participants. Private accounts reflect personal circumstances rather than traditional stereotypes. They reveal the wide range of reflective experiences of ageing and their impact on quality of life. Private accounts comprise complex narrative reconstructions of relationships, events and experience. In explaining these, participants in Corner's study drew on different aspects of their lives as reported in their life histories. Such narratives illustrated how through time the influences of culture and society interacted with personal, emotional, psychological and structural circumstances to elevate important aspects of their lives. Despite the diversity reported by Corner there were areas of similarity and overlap between participants. Thus private accounts high-lighted differences with participants' public accounts as well as differences between private accounts.

In the interpretation of the private accounts of institutionalized ageism Corner (1999) introduced the distinction between three groups of partici-pants: empowered individuals, reluctant collaborators and dominated or oppressed individuals which we discuss in turn shortly. A key factor that helped distinguish these three groups was the sense of control perceived and experienced by study participants. Sense of control is considered to be a critical determinant of psychological well-being and quality of life of older people (Rodin and Langer 1980; Taylor and Ford 1983; Steptoe *et al.* 1991). Control is one important way in which individuals differ and it may be a contributory factor influencing the variability in patterns of adaptation in the context of ageing. When faced with a similar stressor, some people may cope well, whereas others fail to adjust and experience considerable distress. The essential role played by individual control in the lives of older people and their control over life events has been demonstrated in terms of positive outcomes including emotional well-being, successful coping with stress, health outcomes, behaviour change and improved performance (Bandura 1981; Antonovsky 1987). It is also an important aspect of third agers' accounts of a positive quality of life (Blane *et al.* 2002). An appreciation of this concept, therefore, seems important for understanding the meaning of life to older people and for interpreting normal ageing. In Corner's study the dynamics of control were influenced by a number of factors within partici-pants' life histories and were linked to their feelings and experiences of their position as an older person in society. In participants' accounts a sense of change and a sense of dynamism emerged with the inference that control could shift at any time.

For empowered individuals (Corner 1999), control and autonomy was central to their concept of self. They were conscious of the need to manage change and recognized the need to be involved. These individuals were aware that they felt devalued by others 'because they were old' and con-sciously struggled against this using a variety of coping strategies. In their encounters with health and social care professionals and with family and friends they maintained control and successfully negotiated their indepen-dence. In private accounts they challenged institutionalized ageism and demanded that they be treated as individuals with needs in their own right, contradicting the public accounts about ageism.

Reluctant collaborators (Waterworth and Luker 1990; Corner 1999) were frustrated by their inability to influence and control aspects of their lives. But unlike empowered individuals they reluctantly accepted their situations since they perceived there were few other options available to them. They often conformed to the public account while privately holding very different pri-vate views. Throughout their accounts institutionalized ageism was a pivotal theme in defining the quality of their lives. Ageism was experienced in their interactions with health and social care professionals as well as with family and friends.

Dominated or oppressed individuals were more likely to experience overt ageism and infantilization, particularly in their receipt of care. Informal and formal carers adopted a prescriptive approach to care with a rigorous schedule of activities imposed on them. This frequently involved the management of the household as well as providing personal care and prescribed 'treatments'. Control was often seen as having positive intentions:

> He just tries to make life as easy for me as he can. He knows what's best. When I have attacks [angina] he makes me stay in bed, I don't have to, but he says 'stay in bed and have a rest' and then he lets me have a bit potter around ... If I didn't do that I would struggle to do things and so he's bossy for my own good to make sure I don't.
>
> (Corner 1999: 299 [23;6;17])

In these circumstances feelings of disempowerment and helplessness may be a result of low morale associated with the loss of normal health, rather than directly the result of ageism. Chronic illness restricts the choices that are available to healthier older people. But for dominated or oppressed individuals choice was an artificial concept since they did not perceive that there were options open to them. Changes in life conditions and experiences were perceived to be beyond their own control, leading to a state of learned helplessness (Seligman 1992). For many 'convinced that there is no use in responding, these individuals demonstrate motivational deficits such as apathy, listlessness, a decreased incentive to initiate action and "giving up" syndrome' (Seligman 1992).

> I'm dying, I'm so ill, I'm so very ill. I want to die. I don't want to be on this earth any more. I want to die.
>
> (Corner 1999: 303 [25;31;7])

Thus dominated or oppressed individuals' lack of control may lead to learned helplessness that may also reinforce ageism and negative stereotypes of old age. But the fatalism of dominated or oppressed individuals may also underpin different perceptions of 'normal ageing'. Where ageism was perceived as 'normal life' over which they had little control, they appeared to accept this as the status quo. The expectations of normal life were characterized by limited social opportunities and ill health, which in turn would further restrict their social world.

Understanding normal ageing

That ageing is normal is rarely in dispute, since ageing, like birth and death, is a normal experience of human existence. But frequently contested by both natural and social scientists is the idea of 'normal ageing'. Much of the dispute of what is 'normal ageing' is apparently resolved by clarifying the linguistic confusion around the two meanings of the word 'normal'. It can either mean normative or usual, or it can mean non-pathological. For example, cognitive decline is normative in that it is a usual experience of older adults and it increases with increasing age (Rabbitt 1992). While memory loss, mental slowness, anxiety or depression is not uncommon among older people, pathologies such as Alzheimer's disease are not inevitable. Cognitive decline becomes cognitive impairment when impairment of memory plus impairment of at least one other cognitive function is sufficient to interfere with daily activities. Similarly, with regard to normal in the sense of non-pathological, it is extremely rare to find no evidence of Alzheimer's pathology in the brains of non-demented older people (Neuropathology Group of the MRC CFAS 2001). Other pathologies, like osteoporosis, cataract, cancer and hypertension, also provide contested accounts. The prevalence of each of these conditions increases markedly with age.

But has linguistic clarification resolved the contested nature of 'normal ageing'? Biogerontologists have noted that some individuals seem to age fast while others appear to age more slowly. They make the distinction between chronological age, measured by the passage of time, and biological age, measured by biomarkers, for example the level of a blood enzyme (Kirkwood 1999). Although we may contest some claims of extreme longevity, in cultures where past birth and demographic records are of dubious quality, chronological age is relatively easy to determine. But for social scientists, like definitions of pathology and disease, biomarkers remain highly contested. They are a good example of 'boundary work' in science (Gieryn 1983), since they are labels, social constructions determined by scientists and often arbitrary in nature. Hypertension is a classic example of the arbitrary label applied to a 'scientific' measurement. In western societies blood pressure varies between individuals and increases with chronological age. Hypertension is defined by medical convention and people whose blood pressure is above a certain cut-off are labelled hypertensive and may receive treatment. Another example of the arbitrary nature of the boundary between normal and pathology comes from psychiatry. In 1980, the American Psychiatric Association voted to determine whether homosexuality was pathological or normal and decided that it was no longer a psychiatric condition!

So what is the boundary between 'normal ageing' and pathological ageing? We have seen that the process of distinguishing between normal and pathological ageing is grounded in human judgements made by biomedical scientists, rather than scientific facts. And since most chronic conditions become more common with chronological age, the boundary remains highly contested. Much of the debate, however, is confused by differences in the way social scientists and biomedical scientists fashion the debate. The obvious difference is one of focus. Biogerontologists, on the one hand, emphasize biological ageing and concern themselves with establishing biomarkers of the ageing process and identification of factors that account for the considerable variability in human ageing. Social gerontologists, on the other hand, register biological ageing as a social fact and concern themselves in understanding how society, including biomedicine, defines the boundary between normal and abnormal ageing and how boundary definitions affect older people in society.

Common-sense lay knowledge leads many older people to explain biological changes as natural outcomes of the ageing process. The emergence of wrinkles, the balding of heads and the greying of hair are generally accepted as signs of ageing. There is no clear agreement on what constitutes 'normal' ageing in terms of hair loss or natural hair colour. We will have all observed differences in the rate of ageing among our families and friends but such differences are often taken for granted. When we experience a biological change we are likely to attribute the signs to ageing. But the way we each interpret changes in our bodies will reflect the culture, time and place in which we live. 'Personality' may also play a role. Corner (1999) found that study participants who were dominated or oppressed were more likely to attribute 'old age' to many of the medical conditions for which they were being treated. They had a sense of fatalism about their conditions, and a belief that there was little anyone could do for them.

I don't really see there's much they can do really. It's just old age.

I don't think there's anything much they can do. It's just old age.

When you get to my age, there's nothing you can do really.
(Corner 1999: 312 [36;4;19] [19;21;20] [2;13;9])

It is not surprising, therefore, that the underdiagnosis of disease in older people is common. Older people who expect to experience mental and physical symptoms in later life often fail to mention them to their doctors, even when effective treatments exist (Williams 1990).

Of course it is not just older people and other members of the lay public who express such sentiments about 'normal ageing'. Health professionals are equally capable of using old age as an explanation for physical or mental decline. How frequently does one get the response from the doctor that those general aches and pains are 'because of your age'? But sometimes professional expectations may be associated with underdiagnosis, for example the older woman who is told by her doctor that her non-healing broken ankle 'is simply a strain that is slower to heal because you are getting older now and healing is slower at your age'.

Recent developments in treatments for Alzheimer's disease and other types of dementia illustrate how boundary issues between normal and pathological ageing affect the quality of older people's lives. Before 1970 we had little understanding of what caused Alzheimer's disease. Although characterized at the turn of the last century by the psychiatrist Alois Alzheimer it remained classified under the general heading of senile dementia – a classification that associated the vicissitudes of the disease as an almost inevitable consequence of old age. Among many biomedical scientists the boundary between normal and pathological ageing remained blurred and unimportant. Older people with dementia were, prior to 1970, a relatively small group. They were hidden by families and warehoused in the 'asylums' and 'ex-workhouses', invisible not only to the general public but also to the majority of health professionals and biomedical scientists. The quality of the lives of older people living in such institutions has been poignantly portrayed by Townsend (1964) in *The Last Refuge*. His account of a single visit to an ex-workhouse that accommodated older people, including older people with dementia, describes quality of life for older people at the time:

The first impression was grim and sombre. A high wall surrounded some tall Victorian buildings, and the entrance lay under a forbidding arch with a porter's lodge at one side. The asphalt yards were broken up by a few beds of flowers but there was no garden worthy of the name. Several hundred residents were housed in large rooms on three floors. Dormitories were overcrowded, with ten or twenty iron-framed beds close together, no floor covering and little furniture other than ramshackle lockers. The day rooms were bleak and uninviting. In one of them sat forty men in high-backed Windsor chairs, staring straight ahead or down at the floor. They seemed oblivious of what was going on around them. The sun was shining outside but no one was looking that way. Some were seated in readiness at the bare tables even though the midday meal was not to be served for over an hour. Watery-eyed and feeble, they looked suspiciously at our troupe of observers and then returned to their self-imposed contemplation. They wore shapeless tweed suits and carpet slippers or boots. Several wore caps. Life seemed to have been drained from them, all but the dregs. Their stoic resignation seemed attributable not only to infirmity and old age. They were like people who had taken so much punishment that they had become inured to pain and robbed of all initiative. They had the air of not worrying much about their problems because of the impossibility of sorting them out, or the difficulty getting anyone to understand or take notice.

(Townsend 1964: 4)

Recent reports of the quality of life of older people living in institutions in some Eastern European countries mirror this chilling account. In the fifty years, however, since Townsend penned this description, things have improved in the UK for older people resident in long-term care institutions with the building of purpose-built homes, better furnishings and more enlightened caring regimes. That some Victorian workhouses still remain and are used as care homes for older people at the turn of the twenty-first century is deplorable but slowly these are being replaced and demolished. But at the time Townsend was writing there existed an expectation that this was 'normal ageing'. It was not only physical or mental decline that was accepted as normal. It was also the social regimes that existed in these total institutions (Goffman 1961) that were accepted as a normal part of the experience of life for old and frail people.

The rediscovery of Alzheimer's disease during the 1960s and 1970s marked a turning point in the biomedical understanding of 'normal ageing'. The emergence of Alzheimer's disease as a distinct entity was the result of studies identifying the ultrastructure of the plague and tangle in Alzheimer brains at post-mortem in the 1960s and the exciting discovery by groups of independent scientists of the deficit in choline acetyl transferase in the 1970s (Katzman and Bick 2000). This has led to the development of cholinesterase (the enzyme that metabolizes acetylcholine in the brain) inhibitors such as tachrine and donepezil in the treatment of some types of dementia in the 1990s. With the discovery of *a* cause of Alzheimer's disease, cognitive decline was no longer attributed in biomedical science as normal ageing. Rather, because there now existed a potential for a cure, cognitive decline was characterized as pathological ageing. The boundary between normal cognitive decline associated with chronological age and cognitive decline due to Alzheimer's disease and other dementias still remains contested, however, not least because of the recent emergence of mild cognitive impairment (Hogan and McKeith 2001) as a diagnostic label used by psychiatrists to categorize older people with cognitive impairments who may be showing the early signs of a dementing disease (Larrieu *et al.* 2002). The question still persists as to whether cognitive impairment is caused by age or by disease (Holstein 2000), but it remains important to biomedical science that cognitive impairment is understood as pathological because research funding is more widely available to study disease than it is to study normalcy. Alzheimer's disease has become politicized.

In *Oldtimers and Alzheimer's* Gubrium (1986) documents the changing status of Alzheimer's disease and its impact on the social worlds of people with dementia and their informal caregivers. The emergence of Alzheimer's disease changed the status of dementia in the eyes of the public. When it was described as senile dementia it had a low public profile. It was highly stigmatized. Those with dementia were hidden from public and medical view. The new status of Alzheimer's disease is still stigmatized (Bond 2001), but it is more visible and people with Alzheimer's disease receive more sympathy. However, it is the caregivers of people with dementia who have received most sympathy and also recognition for the emotional and physical burden they experience (Aneshensel *et al.* 1995). Increasing the profile of the condition has not been without its cost to the quality of life of people with dementia and their informal caregivers. Few people seek a *cure* for ageing. In scientific and popular culture ageing is inevitable, a part of the human condition. Biomedical research focuses on seeking cures for incapacitating diseases of later life while public concern is around ensuring that we each maintain our quality of life as we age. But the notion that there might be a cure for any disease, perhaps ironically, increases the level of anxiety about the condition. This has certainly been the case for cognitive impairment (Cutler and Hodgson 1996; Hodgson and Cutler 1997; Husband 2000; Alzheimer Scotland – Action on Dementia 2002; Bond and Corner 2002; Corner and Bond 2004). Holstein (2000) reflects on the level of anxiety generated by the politicization of Alzheimer's disease, noting that many physicians in the US describe their patients as 'terrified'. She compares this with the old man Shigezo in Ariyoshi's 1987 novel *The Twilight Years* (Ariyoshi 1987) who does not experience terror as he deepens into profound forgetfulness and incapacity. Rather the novel focuses on the daughter-in-law Akiko's slow transformation of her own busy life to care for her father-in-law. Holstein concludes:

Who is better served – Shigezo or the newly diagnosed patients at a major medical centre? Have we done a disservice to patients and their families by the particular cultural construction of AD that is dominant in American society today? What does this construction suggest about American values, belief systems, and notions about old age? If culture shapes perceptions and understandings of disease, so does disease tell us something important about culture.

(Holstein 2000: 176–7)

Contested accounts of what distinguishes normal and pathological ageing are perhaps not as distinctive as the case of Alzheimer's disease and cognitive impairment, particularly in biomedicine. But the debate around normal ageing and cognitive impairment remains the classic illustration of the difficulties individuals have in understanding their own ageing. And the way that we as individuals perceive normal ageing will have an impact on our own perception of self and our expectations of our quality of life as we age. If we perceive ageing as a process of increasing ill health and disability, of a time of diminished personal and social opportunities, we are likely to accept as inevitable the negative stereotypes of old age and ageism. We are also likely to feel oppressed and dominated and experience a negative quality of life. Those of us who feel in control, who challenge the negative stereotypes of old age and who recognize that many of the biological processes of ageing are not necessarily inevitable are more likely to experience a positive quality of life. This, perhaps too simple, analysis of course assumes that quality of life is a subjective experience, an idea which is highly contested and one which we return to in more detail in the next chapter.

Note

1. Transcript identifier; page number; line number.

5

Explaining quality of life

In their quest to examine aspects of the individual and social ageing, researchers have been quick to provide facts but slow to integrate them within a larger explanatory framework, connecting findings to established explanations of social phenomena.

(Bengston *et al.* 1997: S72)

How much do existing social gerontological theories reflect the concerns and interests of older people? How useful are these theories in explaining the quality of life of older people? In this chapter we will evaluate some of the key theories, which could be used to explain the quality of later life. We do this through a sociological gaze but one that integrates ideas from different perspectives. With few exceptions (Fennell *et al.* 1988), there has not been a consistent attempt within sociology to provide a coherent account of the process of ageing and later life. Feminism (Arber and Ginn 1991; Ray 1996) and the political economy perspective (Townsend 1981; Walker 1981; Estes *et al.* 1982; Phillipson 1982) have provided a sociological gaze on ageing and later life, yet neither account individually or together is entirely satisfactory. The influence of both postmodernism (Fox 1993; Wilson 1995) and social constructionism (Hazan 1994) is implicit in many accounts of ageing, but again neither individually or together provides a satisfactory account of ageing and later life.

Psychologists have taken a different gaze. The study of ageing has had a relatively minor place in psychology (Bond *et al.* 1993). From social psychology, an important contribution has been the life-span perspective (Coleman 1986; Sugarman 1986). From psychology, theories of successful ageing (Baltes and Carstensen 1996) have dominated gerontological writing. These build on a strong US tradition characterized by disengagement theory (Cumming and Henry 1961) and activity theory (Havighurst 1963). But how do these social and behavioural perspectives contribute to our understanding of quality of life? This chapter considers their contributions.

Theories of well-being and life satisfaction

Concern with quality of life did not appear with the creation of the term. Much of the early gerontological work reflected on the personal well-being of older people and satisfaction with their lives. Three of the key and competing theories, which dominated three decades of gerontological research, were activity theory, continuity theory and disengagement theory. In the general gerontological literature these ideas are described as theories, but in the strict sense of the term they are not theories but conceptual frameworks or models made up of loose connections rather than closely argued causal connections. The essence of the activity theory of ageing is that there is a positive rela-tionship between activity and life satisfaction. A linear relationship was postulated: the greater the role loss, the lower the life satisfaction. In contrast, continuity theory emphasizes continuity in people's lives and the strategies of adaptation they use to maintain patterns of thinking, activity profiles, social relationships and overall quality of life. The long-term consistency which is the foundation of continuity theory is not the homeostatic equilibrium predicted by activity theory. Rather, continuity theory sees the relationships between past, present and future patterns of thought, behaviour, social arrangements and quality of life as heterogeneous and flexible. On the other hand, the essence of disengagement theory was the idea that as individuals grow older they and society prepare in advance, by a reduction in social activity and participation, for the ultimate 'disengagement', which is caused by incapacitating disease or death. It assumes that whereas the nature of later life may change, quality of life is maintained because of the individual's preparation for change and the inevitability of disengagement.

Activity theory

The key belief here is that successful ageing can be achieved by maintaining into old age the activity patterns and values experienced in middle age. Happiness in later life is achieved by denying the onset of old age and where the relationships, activities or roles of middle age are lost it is important to replace them with new ones in order to maintain life satisfaction. Support for this theory was found in a number of empirical studies in the US reporting over a twenty-year period between 1950 and 1970. In particular inter-personal activity was found to be consistently important for predicting an individual's sense of well-being in his or her later years. People spending a greater amount of time in social and voluntary organizations were likely to have high personal adjustment (Burgess 1954). High personal morale was found to be strongly associated with high levels of activity (Kutner *et al.* 1956; Reichard *et al.* 1962; Maddox 1963; Graney 1975). High activity levels in advancing age were also found to be good predictors of life satisfaction (Tobin and Neugarten 1961). Relationships with a close confidant have been shown to be protective against depression (Brown and Harris 1978) and to be strongly associated with levels of morale (Lowenthal and Haven 1968). Thus in cross-sectional observational survey data there existed evidence of a relationship between social interaction and activity with what we now call quality of life.

Yet there were few attempts to test formally an explicit activity theory of ageing. A formal exploration of activity theory in relation to different types of activity and life satisfaction found that many of the logical hypotheses for the theory were not supported (Lemon *et al.* 1972). A substantive conclusion was that the simple linear relationship between activity levels and life satisfaction reported in empirical studies was insufficient to explain the complex interaction between individuals and their changing social environments. To the criticism of simplicity can be added one of idealism. It is surely unrealistic to expect the majority of older people to maintain the level of activity and social interaction associated with middle age. Nowadays it may be possible for people in the Third Age to engage in an active lifestyle but for many older people the declines in social networks, loss of close confidants and physical and mental ill health make the maintenance of an active lifestyle a major challenge.

Within social gerontology an activity theory of ageing declined in influence during the last quarter of the twentieth century, although it still has its proponents. The relationship between social activity and quality of life continued to be explored but recent studies have confirmed the complexity of the relationship and the role of environmental and other psychosocial factors (Fernández-Ballesteros *et al.* 2001).

Continuity theory

Continuity theory is a theory of continuous development and adaptation throughout the life course (Atchley 1989). It originated from the observation that despite widespread changes in health status, physical functioning and social circumstances, a large proportion of older people presented considerable consistency in their attitudes and values, patterns of thinking, the kinds of social activities they participated in (Atchley 1998) and the nature of their social networks (Antonucci and Akiyama 1987). Continuity theory builds on these empirical observations to provide an explanation of the long-term consistency in people's lives.

The essence of continuity theory is the ability of people to develop cognitive structures with which they organize and interpret their life experiences (Levinson 1990). As we age, we develop clear conceptions of ourselves and the world around us. We use our lifetime of experiences in patterns of thought to describe and analyse our everyday social world. We make decisions; we act and pursue goals to achieve our daily lives. We are assumed to be dynamic and self-aware entities that know our strengths and weaknesses, what we are capable of, and what we prefer or dislike. Over time we acquire a sense of personal agency. Continuity theory assumes that our patterns of adaptive thought continue to develop through learning across the life course and that the goal is not to remain the same, but to adapt attitudes, values and beliefs in response to life-course change, and social change. Adaptation to life-course and social changes is a process, and necessarily so, because of the inherently conservative nature of human agency (Marris 1986).

The process of lifelong adaptation is influenced by the social context in which we live. Our social constructions of reality (Berger and Luckmann 1966) are influenced by those around us and the mass media. But our own personal constructs (Kelly 1955) develop in response to our life experiences and these determine the way we think about ourselves, our personal lifestyles and quality of life. We are free to decide how we construe our own social reality, however much society tries to influence the way we think about ourselves. This has implications for the way quality of life is defined. Subjective perceptions of our own quality of life will have more significance for theory than so-called objective indicators.

This is not to say that social structure does not influence the development of human agency. The premise of structuralist theories of ageing such as political economy (see below) is that access to material resources, such as education, in the early stages of the life course dramatically influence life-course development and later life experience. Structural characteristics such as gender, ethnicity and social class are important determinants of the experience and quality of life throughout the life course (see Chapter 3). Structural characteristics provide a major continuity in the context of people's lives.

Continuity theory highlights both internal continuity and external continuity. Internal continuity can be assessed in terms of how we maintain a way of thinking about the self and the meaning we give to our lives. External continuity can be observed through the degree of consistency over time of our social roles, activities and relationships, which are the building blocks of our individual lifestyles.

Disengagement theory

In contrast to the activity theory of ageing, disengagement theory was formalized and formally tested in a number of studies. Disengagement theory was first explicated by Cumming and Henry (1961) in *Growing Older:* 'Disengagement is an inevitable process in which many of the relationships between a person and other members of society are severed and those remaining are altered in quality' (Cumming and Henry 1961: 211). The theory states that the process of disengagement is the method by which society prepares for the changing roles of its members so that when the inevitable arrives it does not disrupt the orderly functioning of society.

Conceptually disengagement theory has also been criticized by a number of writers. Three substantial criticisms have been presented. First, by implication the theory suggests that disengagement is desirable and therefore condones a policy of indifference towards the problems of older people (Shanas *et al.* 1968). Second, disengagement is not inevitable and non-engagement in old age reflects the lifelong pattern of social interaction for some people. Third, the data presented in *Growing Older* have been incorrectly interpreted since the cultural values and economic structures themselves lead to a situation in which people not economically active, the majority of older people, are disengaged (Rose 1965). A general conclusion is therefore that 'In the balance, disengagement theory has been found wanting empirically and its original formulation is rarely defended by anyone' (Maddox 1969).

Yet despite the overwhelming negative comment of disengagement theory, its conceptual basis, the idea that older people disengage from active life, remains implicit in some current gerontological theories. Thus like activity theories of ageing it remains too simplistic to account for the complexity of the modern world but is supported by the behaviour of some older people.

Successful ageing

The concept of successful ageing has also been in the gerontological literature for a number of years. Yet it has developed into a more sophisticated idea than that originally described. Earlier uses of the concept were descriptive and related to the idea that successful ageing would be about such factors as good health, economic security and presence of friends and family (Havighurst 1963). But there was disagreement about what constituted a good quality of life. Some believed that a good quality of life consisted of maintaining activity and involvement (activity theory) and others about retirement and release from activities of middle age (disengagement theory). To some extent these early debates have not been satisfactorily resolved. It continues to be used as a descriptor for an idealized quality of later life in contemporary social gerontological writing (Rowe and Kahn 1997; Stevens 2001) But what does constitute successful ageing? Is it simply about satisfaction with life and one's quality of life or does it have a wider use in relation to the impact of ageing on society?

The resurgence of the notion of successful ageing can be attributed to the pioneering work of Baltes and Baltes (1990b). They challenge the traditional social science perspective, which focuses on prescribed outcomes and ideal norms. In contrast, their approach focuses on the processes older people use to achieve desired goals. Rather than measuring successful ageing exclusively in terms of life satisfaction or morale, the traditional approaches used in quality of life research, they focus on understanding the maximization of the benefits associated with ageing together with the minimization of the losses. Their *multicriteria approach* identifies a number of key indicators of successful ageing frequently used to measure outcomes in later life. They argue for a balance between quantitative and qualitative aspects of ageing and propose a number of key indicators (Box 5.1).

This list highlights a challenge for a theory of successful ageing, namely the rivalry between subjective and objective indicators. Baltes and Baltes (1990a) adopt the traditional 'scientistic' position that subjective indicators are unhelpful because of the ability of the human mind to reframe expectations. Objective indicators are therefore seen as the more appropriate. Their critique of subjective indicators focuses on the evidence that people experiencing very different life qualities will report similar views on their quality of life. Nobody living in poverty or people in the dying phase of a terminal illness should express happiness in the same way as someone with all their life to

Box 5.1   Key indicators of successful ageing

- Length of life
- Biological health
- Mental health
- Cognitive efficacy
- Social competence and productivity
- Personal control
- Life satisfaction

Source: Baltes and Baltes (1990b)

live for. However, they recognize the bias of middle-class western values in most of the objective measures used. They therefore concede that both subjective and objective indicators of successful ageing should be considered within a particular social and cultural context. However, indicators alone do not comprise a theory, but rather like earlier theories described above only provide the basis for conceptual models. The theory of successful ageing presented by Baltes and Baltes (1990a) sets out seven propositions. These are shown in Box 5.2. They indicate that this is a psychological theory of successful ageing and many of the propositions are supported by empirical evidence from within psychology. This emphasis therefore 'places sole responsibility for successful ageing on the individual' (Baltes and Carstensen 1996).

Box 5.2   Propositions about human ageing

1   There are major differences between normal, optimal and pathological ageing.
2   There is much variability (heterogeneity) in ageing.
3   There is much latent reserve.
4   There is an ageing loss near limits of reserve.
5   Knowledge-based pragmatics and technology can offset age-related decline in cognitive mechanics.
6   With ageing the balance between gains and losses becomes less positive.
7   The self remains resilient in old age.

Source: Baltes and Baltes (1990a)

Over two decades (Baltes and Baltes 1980, 1990a; Baltes *et al.* 1984; Featherman *et al.* 1990; Baltes and Carstensen 1996) a meta-model of selective optimization with compensation has emerged. In this model success is defined as individual goal attainment and successful ageing as minimization of losses that occur as a result of a reduction in physical, cognitive and social reserves and a maximization of gains that result through adaptation, mastery and the use of wisdom. Three processes have been highlighted: selection, compensation and optimization. An insight into how these processes operate can be gained from the following two examples.

The pianist Rubenstein when asked how he managed to continue playing so successfully at his advanced age responded that he overcame weaknesses in his piano playing by reducing his repertoire and playing a smaller number of pieces (selection); practising these more often (optimization); and slowing down his speed of playing prior to fast movements, thereby producing a contrast that enhances the impression of speed in the fast movements (compensation) (Baltes and Baltes 1990a).

Similarly an older marathon runner can continue to win successfully by competing with his own age group and running fewer and easier courses (selection); varying footwear and extending warm-up periods (compensation) and using a special diet and vitamin supplements to increase fitness (optimization) (Baltes and Carstensen 1996).

The champions of this approach highlight a number of advantages. By taking a process-oriented approach individuals are able to define their own life world and set goals appropriate to their personal needs and desires rather than the imposition of universal social worlds. The approach acknowledges the diversity of older people recognized by earlier generations of gerontologists. 'Age *per se* masks considerable variation in self-conceptions and in the personal and social resources which demonstrably exist among person of the same chronological age' (Maddox 1969). The approach focuses on the individual strategies used to achieve goals rather than simply on outcomes. But centrally this approach focuses on the interplay between gains and losses and provides a positive perspective on human ageing rather than viewing later life as a time of loss, social isolation, impoverishment and dependency.

Over the years the concept of successful ageing has been equated with the idea of a good quality of life. What does the model of successful ageing described above offer individuals who are ageing? A simple six-point guide to successful ageing has been suggested (Box 5.3). But for many individuals such a strategy is not acceptable for social and cultural reasons. Like strategies

Box 5.3   Strategies for successful ageing

1   Engage in a healthy lifestyle to reduce the effects of pathological ageing.
2   Avoid simple solutions and encourage individual and societal flexibility.
3   Strengthen one's reserve capacities through educational, motivational and health-related activities.
4   Identify methods of compensation for limits to reserve capacity through prosthetic devices, age-appropriate lifestyles and age-friendly environments.
5   Assist individuals to acquire effective strategies involving changes in aspirations and the scope of goals.
6   Acceptance of functional and cognitive losses and changes to goals and aspirations.

Source: Baltes and Baltes (1990b)

to improve public health, strategies for improving quality of life through adjustment to the ageing processes would be difficult to implement as public policy. Many of the barriers to adoption of such strategies are the result of the kind of society in which we live. It is to structural theories of ageing, which explain the impact of society on the individual, to which we now turn.

Structural theories of ageing

For a quarter of a century structural theories of ageing have been dominated by the ideas of structured dependency (Walker 1980; Townsend 1981) and the development of the political economy perspective on ageing (Estes 1979; Walker 1981; Estes *et al.* 1982; Phillipson 1982; Minkler and Estes 1999). Political economy is the study of the interrelationships between the political, economic and social structures or specifically relationships between government organizations, the labour market, social classes and status groups. Much of the focus of gerontological theory has been the distribution of social resources in later life. The key concept here is the idea of structured dependency. Structured dependency describes the development of a dependent status resulting from restricted access to a wide range of social resources, particularly income. This is reflected in the large number of older people who are living in poverty (Townsend 1979, 1991; Walker 1993; Atkinson 1995; Johnson and Stears 1997). One in four older people in the UK have incomes which are equal to or below the state poverty line (i.e. eligible for income support) (Walker 1993) (see also Chapter 3). Older women are significantly poorer than their male counterparts (Arber and Ginn 1991). Exit from the labour market is a key explanation of poverty in later life in a society that rewards 'productive' work. But poverty in later life is also strongly related to low resources and restricted access to resources throughout the life cycle (Walker 1993). It is easy to see why. Women comprise the majority of older people. Few of them will have been in full-time employment throughout the adult life cycle. The proportion of older people who were dual earning couples is relatively low (Falkingham and Victor 1991) and the majority of male retirees are low-paid manual workers without adequate occupational pension contributions.

Prior to retirement manual workers experience reduced economic status through unemployment, early retirement and re-employment in less skilled jobs (Townsend 1979; Laczko and Phillipson 1991). After retirement the inequalities resulting from low pay, unemployment and disability and, for women and people from ethnic minority groups, sex and racial discrimination are carried forward into old age. The decline in the real value of savings and pensions means that the worse-off are those who are very old, particularly very old women. Even among younger cohorts of older people the recent increase in housing assets has made minimal improvements to living standards (Hancock 1998). All older people are discriminated against by economic and social policies which benefit the young employed and well off. Retirement also restricts access to social resources in the form of a reduction in social relationships once the retiree is away from the world of work (Phillipson 1982).

The political economy perspective has focused analysis and the development of social explanations on class inequality and the relationship between economic production and later life. In the UK it has been criticized for failing to address issues of gender adequately (Bury 1995). But in the US it has increasingly recognized the strength of the feminist critique and applied the approach to inequalities between men and women in later life and between people from different ethnic groups as well as between different parts of the world. And recently the political economy perspective has examined the impact of globalization on older people (Phillipson 1998; Minkler and Estes 1999). Yet the criticism that the approach is rather narrow (Dant 1988), focusing as it does on inequalities resulting from poverty and economic disadvantage, still holds. The approach has been useful in shifting thinking about status in old age from a negative concentration on individual characteristics to an emphasis on the structural factors which work against older people. But the approach, particularly the notion of structured dependency, is itself capable of reinforcing ageist policy and practice (Wilson 1995).

Structural theories in gerontology have not explicitly addressed quality of life as an issue for older people. The concept is taken for granted with perhaps an implicit assumption that inequality is not only an indicator but also a significant cause of poor life quality. (We examine some of the implicit taken-for-granted assumptions in regard to the status of older people in the UK which underpin this perspective in Chapter 3.) For many the political economy perspective provides a solid base on which to develop an explanation of quality of life in later life. But it does not provide a sufficiently coherent account to explain individual differences in quality of life and, like theories of successful ageing, highlights the centrality of objective indicators like inequality and deprivation without taking sufficient account of older people's self-identity.

Self in society

The traditional contest between individual- or micro- and societal- or macro-level explanations are increasingly being set aside within social gerontology with attempts to integrate self and society or identity and structure in gerontological theory (Ryff and Marshall 1999). That self or identity should be considered as an outcome of social structures is not a new idea (Cooley 1902). Likewise the perspective that individuals create and change society is equally not new (Mead 1934). Also it is now well recognized that the nature of self and identity are influenced by both time and place and are therefore historically and culturally relative (Neisser and Jopling 1997). Similarly we would argue that quality of life is defined by an individual's own sense of self and identity. Both subjective personal experience and objective social circumstances mould the nature of self. Thus given the very different and heterogeneous life-course experiences of older people from different cultures and subcultures across time and space it is the very nature of self which determines the meaning that any individual gives to his or her own quality of life.

Thus in order to understand the meaning of quality of life we need to examine our sense of self or personal identity. Our sense of self emerges from a number of interactive elements of our social and psychological experience (Gecas and Burke 1995: 42). First, a sense of self develops through situated interactions across the life course. The primary components of the life course are an individual's interactions with 'others' in the external world. An 'other' may be a person, a social group, an institution or culture, or a particular object or place (Levinson 1990). Second, a sense of self will be mediated by the structural nature of the person's social roles and social group processes. How others perceive one's identity will impact on the sense of self. Here an important distinction is between the self of personal identity in which one's sense of personal agency supports continuity of purpose and meaning in life and the sense of self that persists 'behind' what Goffman called 'personae', this is the self which is publicly displayed in everyday interaction (Goffman 1971). Third, personal experiences situated in time and place will influence the development of a sense of self. For current generations of older people the experience of living through the Great Depression of the 1930s and World War II (1939–45) has influenced many older identities while for others the loss of parents early in life may have challenged their sense of self in later life (Brown and Harris 1978). Fourth, intrapersonal processes linked to biological and psychological processes will influence the development of a sense of self through ontogenetic changes across the life course, for example progressive intellectual growth leading to wisdom in later life. Finally, the sense of self will be contingent on the interaction of available personal resources and social capital within the context of an individual's social world (Hendricks 1999). It is the context of that social world to which we now turn.

Modernism and postmodernism

The latter half of the twentieth century saw the transition from modernity through late modernity (Giddens 1991) to a postmodern society (Bauman 1992). Characteristics of this process include the increasing interdependence of world societies through the process of globalization. This has been an uneven and fragmented process, which has highlighted and accelerated inequalities between different regions of the world and reinforced the hegemony of transnational corporations within the world economy. The innovation of telecommunication technologies and advances in transportation have facilitated global communication and rapid exchange of goods between different parts of the world (Giddens and Birdsall 2001). Globalization has been accompanied by more flexible forms of work organization, the disruption to family and kinship networks, the blight of local communities and the weakening of the institutions and practices of the state (Phillipson 1998). For individuals the change towards a postmodern world is about living in a world where traditional routines and institutions are abandoned. In the postmodern world we are charged with the task of negotiating new lifestyles and making new choices about how to live our lives (Giddens 1991). This changing social context has significant impact on life quality and how we define our sense of self.

The self in a postmodern world

A key issue for the postmodern citizen is the consumer culture and the way many individuals present themselves through the ubiquitous process of consumption. Consumption is one way in which the postmodern self can express its self-identity. Indeed, one would think from the writings of some postmodernists on the one hand, and the incessant advertising of new consumer products on the other hand, that the only way to express self-identity is through conspicuous consumption. One driver of social change over the last fifty years has been the emergence of the 'affluent society' (Galbraith 1962). One predicted consequence of the affluent society was the increase in leisure time across the life course. That those in paid work appear not to have experienced an increase in leisure time is just one of the predictions signalled by Galbraith's polemic that have not yet come to fruition. But 'the affluence of large parts of the population has fuelled the idea that identity can be constructed and consumed' (Gilleard and Higgs 2000: 25). Consequently, in life after paid work, the status attributed to an individual may no longer be central to self-identity. Rather self-identity is expressed, revised and represented through patterns of consumption. Thus retirement from paid work represents both a distinct post-work stage in the life course and an expanded opportunity for consumption and new later life opportunities (Gilleard and Higgs 2000: 28–58). Of course, this raises the partly moral question as to whether conspicuous consumption necessarily leads to a higher quality of life – an empirical question, for which there does not appear to a satisfactory answer.

The notion that consumerism is the key driver in the construction of personal identities in later life is perhaps oversimplistic, exploiting the atheoretical position of the sociology of postmodernity (Bauman 1988). We suspect that for many past work status still remains an important driver of self-identity in later life. But there is no dispute that increasing diversity in later life, reflecting the diversity of experience across the life course of men and women, people of different cultures and ethnic traditions and people from different generations, will be reflected in the variety of self-identities constructed by individuals and in the way these are presented within postmodern society. In addition, and perhaps of increasing significance given recent world events, has been the importance of spirituality in self-identity in later life and its influence on quality of life (see Chapter 2).

Self-identity and quality of life

Our review of social and behavioural science theory leads us to the conclusion that the key to understanding quality of life and an individual's evaluation of his or her own quality of life is strongly influenced by an individual's own sense of self or self-identity. Indeed, we would hypothesize that individuals exhibiting a positive sense of self are those who evaluate their quality of life positively, an idea which is not new (Schwartz 1975). We would also conclude that self-identity will take many diverse forms influenced not just by the dominant consumer culture of our postmodernist world but by individuals' life course experience and their current life circumstances as well as the context of social structures with which they engage. However, the links between evaluations of quality of life and self-identity are subjective and subject to considerable personal reflexivity, making this a difficult hypothesis to test within the positivist research paradigm.

By claiming that quality of life is a subjective state we set aside a tranche of theoretical work that conceptualizes quality of life as having objective status. As Andrews and Withey (1976) observed in their analysis of social indicators of well-being, there is little mileage in contesting the pros and cons of objective and subjective measures since to some extent all human evaluations are subjective. Rather we have chosen to locate quality of life as central to the individual human existence, indeed to the individual's sense of self or self-identity. But equally important is our conviction that we cannot conceptualize the quality of life of the self in isolation from the wider social world. Objective and other structural factors will therefore provide both the context and the antecedents of an individual's quality of life. The fascination for us is how they interrelate with one another. We return to these ideas in our final chapter. But first we need to consider how quality of life is measured. This we do in the next chapter.

6

Assessing quality of life

> Quality of life ... is implicit and highly subjective and seems to be a concept that is hard to express as a quantity.
>
> (Leplege and Hunt 1997: 47)

How do we know what is important to someone's quality of life? We have seen in previous chapters that quality of life is extremely difficult to define and therefore it is perhaps unsurprising that it is considered equally challenging to assess or measure. What makes one person's quality of life better or worse than another? How can this be assessed? Who is best suited to judge? The answer to these questions is certainly subjective: what one person cites as being important to their quality of life may be very different to another person's and this may change over time. In this chapter, we will review the key issues in assessment of quality of life in gerontological research, which has been dominated in recent years by 'health-related quality of life'. We will compare different methods used routinely in research and discuss some of the conceptual, theoretical and practical issues of assessing and measuring quality of life. We will also explore why quality of life is a central outcome in gerontological research and discuss the importance of gaining the perspective of the older person.

Epistemologies underpinning quality of life assessment

We have seen in Chapter 5 that much of the work on quality of life assessment emerged from early psychological and sociological approaches to life satisfaction and happiness exploring what makes 'life good' (Neugarten *et al.* 1961; Gubrium and Lynott 1983). These studies retain enormous contemporary relevance, not least because they deal with fundamental questions about the different influences on a person's life which gives it quality. In assessing quality of life, the terms 'successful ageing', 'well-being', 'positive ageing' and 'life satisfaction' continue to be used as a proxy for quality of life (Bowling and Browne 1991; Bowling and Farquhar 1991). Quality of life assessment is now a major industry. During the last two decades of the twentieth century the concept has had a meteoric rise as evidenced by books on quality of life measures (Qureshi 1994; Bowling 1995a, 1996). There are internet websites (www.qolid.org), a professional society, the International Society of Quality of Life Research, and new texts and articles appearing weekly in academic books and journals. It now spans an enormous array of concepts. It is a multidisciplinary enterprise which brings together the perspectives of sociologists, psychologists, philosophers, clinical and social scientists, statisticians and economists. The multidisciplinary nature of quality of life enquiry means that depending on which perspective you take, you will have a preference for how to assess it and what to measure. An oncologist, for example, may be interested in a patient's evaluation of his or her chemotherapy treatment. By contrast, to a town planner quality of life might represent the availability of parks and green, open, undeveloped spaces.

Identifying and understanding what is important to a person's quality of life is an extremely complex process in itself and translating this data into more practical issues of measuring quality of life is fraught with difficulty. Optimism about the *potential* of measuring quality of life has consistently run up against the problem of the lack of *evidence* that quality of life tools are actually measuring what they purport to. A number of different conceptual approaches to quality of life have contributed to current understanding and to the way in which efforts are made to measure it. Considerable ambiguity exists about both the purpose and methods of quality of life assessment. There is now an enormous array of questionnaires (also called instruments or measures) which have been developed for quality of life assessment. The main rationale for their development has been recognition of the need to include the person's perspective as it is widely acknowledged that their views may differ from those of researchers. They vary widely in their intended purpose, content, length, form of delivery and measurement properties. However, despite numerous attempts to define and conceptualize the term quality of life, there is still little consensus over definitions and terminology and it remains a vague, multidimensional concept (Bowling 1995c; Bowling *et al.* 2003). There is still no clear definition about what constitutes quality of life and what affects it. Conceptual confusion is exacerbated by confusion between terms such as quality of life, health-related quality of life, health status and well-being. This presents very real theoretical, practical and methodological challenges to measurement. However, with a few exceptions (Leplege and Hunt 1997) there has been little discontent, within health services research for example, with the dominant paradigm, which uses positivist methods, and the normative approaches associated with it remain largely unquestioned. This is explored in the next section.

The normative approach and positivism

The dominant perspective in assessing quality of life is the narrative 'expert' approach and positivism. The methods of the natural sciences and positivism in social science are the products of the Enlightenment, an eighteenth-century movement based on notions of human progress through the application of reason and rationality. A key tenet of positivism is that all scientific knowledge should be acquired in the same manner. Quantitative methods became the substantive approach to method for much of the social sciences. A criticism of such an approach is that this affinity to the methods of the natural sciences reduces social science to a technical enterprise which has no necessary value implications. Yet, within the social sciences, positivism has been the centre of heated debate. The challenge to positivism and the quantitative approach to method came from a number of directions in social science, from symbolic interactionism, phenomenology and ethnomethodology and increasingly from feminism and postmodernism. Phenomenology and ethnomethodology rejected positivism and quantitative methods from a substantially methodological perspective rather than the theoretical stance of feminism and postmodernism. Positivist approaches are forced to make judgements about which topics to select to deal with, and to categorize and sub-divide topics – pigeon holing responses.

The normative approach to defining and assessing quality of life, rooted in functionalist social science, is driven by the values and perspectives of the people who developed the instruments or measures – generally younger, middle-class professionals or researchers. Normative methods entail a uniform method of data collection which enforces a particular mode of description and classification on the 'reality' being studied. Typically, standardized instruments or measures have been developed to measure quality of life whether using single questions or multi-item scales. These methods also emphasize the psychometric properties of measures, specifying appropriateness, reliability, validity, responsiveness to change, precision, interpretability, acceptability and feasibility. What is meant by these terms is addressed by all the standard textbooks on outcome measurement in health care (McDowell and Newell 1987; Bowling 1996) and is summarized in Table 6.1.

Objectivity versus subjectivity

Scientific rationality assumes there is one true reality which can be discovered if only researchers are objective enough. This pursuit of objectivity has, in part, been influenced by the need of social scientists to attain the status accorded to those working in the natural sciences (Giddens 1976). Initial attempts to measure quality of life focused on *objective* indicators, such as material welfare and levels of income, education and housing (see Chapter 3). In health care settings, clinicians, for example, use a variety of biomedical tests or indicators, such as blood pressure, blood tests, urine tests and x-rays. These data are generally seen as objective, measurable and readily comparable across a range of locations (McColl *et al.* 1997). In reality, quality of life is a collection of interacting objective and subjective dimensions. Baltes and

Table 6.1 Questions that need to be asked of any quality of life measure

Appropriateness	Is the measure relevant to the person or the intervention proposed?
Acceptability	Will the person find the measure acceptable?
Reliability	Are the items measured consistent with each other? Is any bias introduced by the use of one or more raters? Are the results reproducible on repeated administration?
Validity	Does the measure cover all the experiences of the person? Does the measure relate to other theoretically linked variables?
Responsiveness	Does the measure detect relevant changes over time?
Precision	Does the measure cover the whole range of outcomes or does it have ceiling and floor effects?
Interpretability	Is it clear what any resulting numerical value represents?

Baltes (1990a) have argued that quality of life should only be measured in objective terms and that subjective experience and subjectivity are weak concepts.

Quality of life domains

There is now a considerable literature highlighting what is important to older people's quality of life (see Chapter 2). The subjective experience and wider contextual factors seem critical to our understanding of quality of life. These include the physical and social environment; socio-economic and cultural factors; personality factors; personal autonomy factors; subjective well-being; health status and clinical characteristics. We have also seen that the factors that older people highlight as important to their quality of life are the same as other groups. These broadly include relationships with family and friends, social contacts, own health, independence, mobility, emotional well-being, material circumstances, religion/spirituality, leisure activities and the home environment (Farquhar 1994). Social environmental factors such as social integration, the importance of having a purpose in life and belonging to a community have all been identified as being important to quality of life (Qureshi *et al.* 1998; Bamford and Bruce 2000). Other factors which are well covered in the gerontological literature include self-esteem (Coleman 1984), a sense of self and identity (Tobin and Liebermann 1976), a sense of control (Rodin and Langer 1980) and spiritual well-being (Riley *et al.* 1998). These concepts are important in giving people a positive view of themselves and impact on their relationships with friends and families and their activities. They are also important to their continuing ability over the life course to manage their lives, adapt to changes and see meaning in their lives (Fry 2000). However, these concepts have been largely ignored in the measurement of quality of life of older people in health care settings, which have tended to focus on narrow, medically orientated definitions of health. A key to understanding quality of life is to illustrate the interactions between the different domains, contextualized within different individuals' life biographies.

The individual's perspective on quality of life

Quality of life through the gaze of older people is very different from that seen through the gaze of researchers and other so-called experts. Understanding people's individual values and the judgements they make is crucial to understanding their perception of their quality of life. Each person has a unique perspective on what is important to his or her quality of life over time. We could suggest that it is the *meaning* that an individual attaches to an event or series of events that is significant. People can only articulate their subjective experience, in line with their own personal beliefs, views and experiences, contextualized in their own social world and circumstances. Only they can say what they consider to be a 'normal' range of experience, and, theoretically, only they can say how they are affected. The 'individual' view, then, may be different to the 'expert' or 'professional' view.

Through the gaze of the 'expert', quality of life can become something rather different. An analogy can be made here between the different lenses of medicine and social science as focused at disability. The medical gaze, with its emphasis on physical impairment and the need for a medical response, underpins services for older people and is part of the underlying philosophy behind the development of the majority of outcome measures, including quality of life. Thus quality of life measures used in health care settings have tended to focus on narrow, medically orientated definitions of health. People who identify 'social integration' as an important aspect to their quality of life, or whose greatest anxiety is the effect of their illness on their spouse do not fit the traditional medical approach to measurement of health-related quality of life.

This contrast between the 'expert' or professional definitions of quality of life and the lay perspective is therefore very important in the assessment of quality of life. The key features of the medical model may not be the distinction between disease or disability but rather the fact that the medical profession, in the context of health and in other walks of life, has been given the authority, legitimated by society (Freidson 1975), to define quality of life. Issues surrounding the 'measurement' of quality of life have come about as powerful groups dominate our 'scientific thinking'. Of course, in this context, social gerontologists are an expert group imposing their definitions of quality of life on older people, who have their own lay perspective. However, older people are also 'experts' on their quality of life.

Health-related quality of life

The emphasis on satisfaction with life among older people has been superseded in recent decades by a focus on quality of life in *health* and *health care*. In order to distinguish between quality of life in the broader sense, and the requirements of clinical medicine, the term 'health-related quality of life' is now widely used. Bowling (1996) comments that in health research it is increasingly fashionable to equate all non-clinical data with 'quality of life', though few in fact undertake a comprehensive quality of life assessment. A major difficulty for quality of life enquiry is that we may be attempting to quantify quickly what is not easily amenable to quantification. Outside laboratory settings and highly controlled experimental studies, there are major difficulties in controlling for confounding factors, such as environmental and social conditions, and therefore attributing any change to a specific intervention is extremely problematic. There can be a number of influences on a person's health, only some of which are related to the care received (McColl *et al.* 1997). For example, someone might indulge in risk-taking behaviour despite information provided about that risk.

The emergence of health-related quality of life as a dominant theme in gerontological research largely reflects three broad trends. First, there has been a shift in medical preoccupation from the management of acute conditions to chronic disease. For the majority of people with chronic illness, a significant proportion of whom are older people, a cure is not a realistic option and the aim of health care becomes to manage care, to slow the natural progression of disease and maintain life quality. Second, information on health outcomes, including health-related quality of life, is required by all levels and sectors of the health and social services as a means of assessing and comparing the effectiveness and efficiency of new and existing interventions and health technologies. For individual clinicians outcome measurement is an integral part of routinely monitoring the progress of individual patients and is used to establish a reliable basis for clinical decision making. Outcome measurement is also high on the research agenda. Third, widespread changes in the structure and management of the NHS and in health care in the UK have been accompanied by conscious attempts by government to shift power from the medical profession to a managed business culture with emphasis on the perspective of the individual, variously termed the patient, consumer, user, customer or client. The expectation has been that users of health and social care services should be involved in decisions about how we judge the efficiency and effectiveness of services within a democratic system. A consequence of this rhetoric is the notion that if individuals are encouraged to participate in decision-making processes this will lead to a focus on what is important to them and the identification of effective outcomes, which are relevant and appropriate to different individuals and those caring for them.

Being able to assess quality of life in health care settings, then, potentially has many uses. Quality of life assessments are now seen as relevant to clinical decision making in that they provide information about the degrees to which disease and the treatment of disease enhance or detract from a person's ability to function physically, socially and psychologically. Quality of life assessments may be helpful in making judgements about health technologies, such as organ transplantations, which raises ethical and moral questions as to what kind of life is being prolonged. They also play a role in the examination of costs and benefits of alternative treatments – different drugs, for example, or services, in the context of public debate about the allocation of limited resources. They may also be used to make comparisons between disease groups. However, there are dangers of using outcome measures, including quality of life measures, in these different ways. There are now so many different measures on the market that selecting which quality of life measure to use can be a bamboozling choice. Many instruments, even those with a 'track record', are sometimes used in inappropriate situations or under conditions in which the instrument could not be reasonably expected to give a useful and reliable answer. Consequently, this could mean costly resources are used on a useless data collection exercise and people using the measures may have difficulties in the administration, analysis or interpretation of data. 'Most dangerously, inappropriate choice and application of measures may yield an apparently plausible, yet fundamentally flawed answer, leading to inappropriate decisions and actions for patients, health services or society at large' (McColl *et al.* 1997: 12).

Quality of life in outcome research

How quality of life for individuals changes over time is extremely important in health outcome research. In policy research, including health, an outcome is the attributable effect, or lack of effect, of an intervention. The key point is *proof of attribution* – how to determine whether changes, usually measured at different points in time, are the result of the intervention or whether they would have happened anyway – a cause–effect relationship. A potential difficulty is that users of the quality of life instrument may *assume* that because of their intervention quality of life is automatically improved. For example, if a drug was given to a person with Alzheimer's disease and this drug was intended to improve memory, is it an automatic assumption that quality of life is improved because memory has improved? This may be the case, but there may be many other factors influencing that person's quality of life, and improved memory may be only one of them. A potential difficulty for clinicians in assessing quality of life in health care is that because of the nature of their job, they often only see older people with that particular condition. It is perhaps understandable to assume, therefore, that the consequence of that disease is the most important factor affecting the quality of life of their patient and that by treating the disease or symptoms they will improve quality of life. However, health is only one aspect of quality of life and we know from the numerous studies conducted on living with chronic illness and ageing in general that people may adapt and manage any changes in their life as part of what they perceive as normal ageing (see Chapter 4). Their illness, while important, is only one of many important events that have happened over the life course.

We can illustrate this by the following example. Mrs Kennedy (a pseudonym) had arthritis in her knee. She was receiving physiotherapy and as a result she felt that her mobility had improved. However, she had found climbing the stairs in her house extremely difficult and had fallen on several occasions, injuring her back. Social services had subsequently arranged for her to move to a ground floor flat, which was located on the edge of a large 'problem' estate, several miles away from her previous home and friends and family. Mrs Kennedy felt extremely vulnerable and reluctant to leave her house, especially after dark. Far from facilitating greater independence, this move had actually left her feeling 'worse off'. She felt her health had improved over the last month, but that her quality of life had deteriorated as this extract from an interview with her illustrates:

You expect a fair bit of problems health wise when you get older, it's
relatively normal isn't it? . . . The treatment on the knee has helped me, I
do feel I can move around and that, but I feel trapped in these four walls.
I feel more down now than I ever was when the knee was bad . . . My
quality of life is much worse than it was back then.

(Corner 1999: 263)

Traditional approaches to the assessment of quality of life ignore the
symbolic nature and *meaning* of life to the individual. They assume that
individual perceptions remain unchanged. Where changes are recognized
they are treated technically in terms of 'response shift' (Schwartz and
Sprangers 1999). But quality of life is a personal and fluid concept. It is well
illustrated from models of chronic illness how people adjust and cope with
illness (Gubrium 1987; Radley and Green 1987; Anderson and Bury 1988;
Bury 1991; Charmaz 2000). What is important to stress is that these illnesses
are incorporated into people's lives, as another factor over the life cycle. The
process of adaptation is dynamic. Encouraging participants to discuss these
issues in a research context may have implications for people's perception of
their everyday life. By getting people to think through, conceptualize and
articulate their views and beliefs, researchers have to recognize that they may
be a part of a process that changes individuals' expectations, judgements they
make and the meaning that their circumstances have for them. This may
present particular ethical, moral and methodological challenges as to how
this is managed within research practice. People's experiences mean that
their perceptions, their relationships and roles all change over time and
approaches to assessing quality of life need to consider how these huge
variations in values and perceptions and rates of adaptation can be incorporated.

Traditional approaches are grounded in the researcher's definition of the
situation and the extent to which this is shared by participants is unknown
because of the nature of 'public accounts' (Cornwell 1984) (see Chapter 2).
Individualized approaches to measurement of quality of life have been
developed to address some of these challenges (O'Boyle *et al.* 1994; Ruta *et al.*
1994). These approaches enable individuals to identify domains which are
important to their quality of life without being constrained by individual
questions. However, responses may be initially sought with qualitative
methods but the original meaning of what the person said may be lost as
analysis reduces answers to tick boxes, checklists etc. – a process which has
been criticized for 'pigeon-holing' responses.

Although these often frustrate practical men and women who would
like to see all research findings reduced to checklists, bullet points or
score cards for action, they are fundamental to understanding the limits
of confidence to our ability to have knowledge of and act upon the world
around us.

(Murphy *et al.* 1998: 55)

To illustrate these points, we present two brief case studies of two older
people (Corner 1999; Bond *et al.* 2002). Names are pseudonyms.

Case study 1: Mrs Gaynor

A widow for fifteen years, she lived in a quiet street in a terraced house some distance from the main road. She now only lived in the downstairs of the house as she could not manage the stairs. The lounge at the front of the house had been converted into a bedroom: the dining room at the back had become the lounge. Her son lived in Canada and, while they spoke weekly on the phone, he did not visit regularly. She was a slight woman, very slender, about five feet tall and walked with a slight stoop. She enjoyed reading but her eyesight had deteriorated and she was now unable to read for long periods of time. Before she retired, Mrs Gaynor had worked in a material shop for twenty years, while her husband was an engineer at a local chemical plant. She was 92.

Mrs Gaynor described herself firmly during an interview as 'fully independent'. Prior to attending the day hospital she had not been out of the house for six months. A home help brought her shopping and collected her pension and frozen meals were delivered daily. She heated these herself. So long as she was able to do this, she considered herself independent. She also felt she had some control over her life, in that she was living in her own home. She both expected and accepted that certain tasks, such as shopping, would be carried out for her as she felt some decline in her physical activity was an inevitable part of the ageing process:

> Well, you expect it at my age, of course. I don't think I do bad, actually
> ... although I'm very unsteady on my feet and I can't walk far now.
> (Corner 1999: 243)

Mrs Gaynor was questioned about the fact that she had not left the house for six months and how this affected her quality of life. She said that she especially missed not being able to go to the library as reading was still her great passion and she had to rely on what friends brought her which limited both her choice and amount of reading material. This wish to 'get out more' was seized upon by the team at the local day hospital, who immediately prioritized improving Mrs Gaynor's mobility and arranged for her to receive physiotherapy for six weeks. If her arthritis was treated, they argued, her mobility would improve and Mrs Gaynor could once again 'get out more' which would improve her quality of life. However, over the course of interviews, Mrs Gaynor suggested that this solution was not as simple as it would appear. The local bus stop was a ten-minute walk from her house, the pavements were cracked and she felt she had lost confidence and was now frightened of falling. Because of changes to the local bus services she now had to change buses to reach the library and as there was no seat at the bus stop she felt that she could not stand while waiting for the next bus. She could not afford a taxi and friends did not have transport to give her a lift.

Mrs Gaynor did not perceive her illness or mobility problems alone prevented her from actively participating in activities. For example, until six months ago, she had enjoyed attending her local church. She cited her religion as an important aspect of her quality of life. The church was located 500 metres from her house, up a steep incline which she could not walk up. Her ability to get to church on her own was therefore restricted in some respects due her physical condition. However, she felt that the real barrier was not *her* limitations but rather the limitation of her circle of friends, or at least these factors in combination. Without anyone to volunteer to help her into a car and drive her to church she was unable to attend.

This example illustrates how many factors in addition to her health problems militate against Mrs Gaynor 'going out more'. Environmental, transport and financial issues are all important contributory factors to her achieving quality of life in this instance and focusing on one factor at the expense of other factors means that we do not fully understand quality of life from her perspective. A narrow focus on health alone can mask wider contextual factors which are equally important to understanding what gives her life quality. Equally, to another person, especially perhaps a younger person, not leaving the house for six months would be unthinkable. Yet Mrs Gaynor had adapted so that this had become 'normal' to her and she was adamant that it did not bother her unduly. A number of factors can be identified as being important to this including personality traits and life biography. To an outsider some people may appear hugely disadvantaged and incapable of performing tasks for themselves, but they may still retain a sense of control over their circumstances and, importantly, change in their circumstances which contributes to their sense of well-being and overall to their perceived quality of life.

Case study 2: Margaret and Dennis

Margaret and Dennis had been married for 35 years. They lived in a modern terrace of housing, which had been adapted to suit Margaret's needs. She had severe arthritis and oedema in her legs and while she could walk around the house with two sticks, she found it difficult to get up from a chair alone and had had a stair lift fitted. With the use of an electric wheelchair she remained independent. Dennis was an athlete and keen gardener. His physical build was lean and slight and it was not hard on meeting him to imagine him pounding the pavements pursuing his passion for long distance running. For over thirty-five years he had been an active member of a local running club, training with fellow members for marathons, completing daily training runs and exercising in the gym. Through the running club, he ran competitively throughout his long career, completing over twenty-five half marathons and, the crowning of his achievements, completing a local marathon in 3 hours, 10 minutes. The running club also constituted a major part of his social life. He and fellow members met once a week in a local pub and he had developed many close friendships with other club members. Running was clearly important to his quality of life and to his sense of identity. Keeping physically fit was also hugely important to him. He eloquently described the sense of freedom he had always felt when running, how he found running relaxing and how he cleared his mind, running on 'auto-pilot'. The sense of achievement he felt when completing a run was 'fantastic':

> Your body feels good all the time, that's what it feels like, it drives you on because you are wanting to do that all the time and get faster.
>
> (Interview 2, page 19, line 18)

This passion and enthusiasm only came to light following a chance remark by his wife, when discussing 'days gone by' in a qualitative interview. When questioned specifically about what was important to their quality of life, neither raised the topic. It was only after several meetings that the topic came to light.

Dennis had been experiencing memory problems for six years when he was diagnosed with probable Alzheimer's. Almost immediately following this diagnosis Dennis withdrew from running. Friends from the local club no longer contacted him to join them. This had been particularly hurtful to Dennis and he had felt unable to contact his friends, and his closest friend in particular, for an explanation as to why the contact had ceased. Margaret explained:

> ... a friend of his, a very good friend actually, they've been running for years together, came out and saw him last year and said 'Right, Dennis, I'm still running ... I'll come and pick you up and I'll take you and I'll bring you back, give us a ring if you want to go.' So, I says 'Do you want to go?' 'Yes.' So I rang and told him he wanted to go and he never rang back and that really, really upset him. I don't think he ever got over that yet.
>
> (Interview 1, page 9, line 1)

Margaret, described the effect that this incident had had on Dennis:

> I think he's frightened of getting let down again, you know ... he's frightened to trust again.
>
> (Interview 1, page 9, line 27)

Margaret felt Dennis could no longer go out running, focusing on the risks involved and the potential consequences. She expressed her fear of him being hurt, getting lost and being unable to find his way home. Dennis no longer goes out running. He said that he wished he could still run, and felt that he still could. Physically he remains fit and lean; still the body of an athlete. But others have placed restrictions on his choices.

No attempt was actually made to facilitate him pursuing his enjoyment of running. For example, there is an enclosed park nearby. Others deemed this an 'unacceptable risk'. Professionals legitimized the caregiver's feelings, and no attempts were made to take on board just how important running was to Dennis's self-concept. This emphasis on the dementia and the losses had had a huge effect on his quality of life, and a catastrophic effect on how he perceived himself.

Dennis and Margaret were both keen gardeners. Dennis had always enjoyed pottering in the garden, but the pleasure from what was once a particularly enjoyable activity has been diminished by the fact that he now feels 'hemmed in' in the garden. He still feels he has a lot of energy, 'always on the go', and energy that he once diverted into running has nowhere to be channelled, leaving him feeling frustrated and empty.

> He's like a bear with a sore head if he can't get outside. Paces the floor and drives me mad because ... if he's in the house he's on top of me all the time.
>
> (Interview 3, page 10, line 51)

These case studies are intended to illustrate how an understanding of a person's life biography is crucial to understanding what is important to and influences their quality of life. Health issues, in the latter study Dennis's dementia, are one factor over the life course. Each individual is involved in meaningful relationships with others in an often complex network of interactions and social networks (Wenger and Jerrome 1999). Separating health from these broader contextual factors is artificial and severely impairs the validity of any measurement tool.

Challenging quality of life assessment

This chapter has outlined some of the key influences on assessing quality of life to date. We have attempted to illustrate some of the barriers to traditional quality of life assessment using examples from our research on the health of older people and their experience as users of health services. We have shown that there are many influences on a person's quality of life in addition to health over the life course. Methods to capture quality of life in gerontological studies need to examine quality of life within the *context* of the relationship between the individual and society. Although quality of life is a subjective, personal experience, a narrow focus on the individual at the expense of wider contextual factors may be detrimental. Perhaps the key challenge is to develop more innovative and pluralistic approaches to quality of life assessment to try and capture the information from the person, while meeting the needs of professionals who argue for a way of detecting changes in quality of life as a key element of research and practice. Yet, critics of existing approaches argue that current approaches fail to identify *priorities* and the *meaning* of domains to a person's quality of life. Existing measures may be limited in that they do not capture all the dimensions relevant to quality of life, their complexity or how these factors interact within a social, political and economic context. The term quality of life remains useful as an 'indicator' of what is important, but whether we can truly measure quality of life remains extremely uncertain. Thus 'Quality of life may offer us a "sensitising concept" for thinking through the purpose and methods of human services, or ways to enhance the "liveability" of our particular communities in a democratic, inclusive and "emancipatory way" '(Rapley 2003: 212).

7

Rethinking quality of life

'Quality of life' deployed as an official or technical term, operates in
the same manner as all other social-scientific terms. That is it cannot
but homogenize that which it intends (and claims) to pick apart.
(Rapley 2003: 216–17)

This book has been a challenge to write, not least in presenting our view,
which along with a number of others begins to contest the usefulness of
quality of life as a term and concept in understanding the social world of
older people. As we have seen, a term that at the outset seems relatively
simple and self-explanatory is as complex as many other social science ideas.
Within the confines of six chapters we have examined quality of life and the
relevance of the concept to older people. Our treatment could not be
exhaustive and we have therefore been selective in our choice of material.
This chapter brings together a number of the issues explored in earlier
chapters. From Chapter 1 we note the politicized context of the variety of
meanings and uses of quality of life as a social science term and concept. It is
in Chapter 1 that we first highlight the distinction between the 'objectivity' of
quality of life as 'measured' by the social indicators movement and the
'subjectivity' of the lived experience of older people. Our emphasis is one of
the relative nature of quality of life and the importance of taking the perspective of the other. Chapter 2 presents accounts of how older people think
about quality of life and what a good life means to them. We present both
their public and private accounts using a framework suggested by the findings of Bowling and Windsor (2001), Bowling (1995b, 1995c) and Farquhar
(1994, 1995). We use a social indicator approach in Chapter 3 to place the
rich accounts of older people within the socio-economic context of older
people in twenty-first-century Britain, a context that many older people
accept and take for granted, perhaps reflecting their lack of consciousness of

their oppressed status in contemporary society. The ideas of Chapter 4 focus on the way older people are represented in everyday life and the way we think about ageing. This provides the socio-cultural context in which older people live out their lives and which is a potent influence on the quality of their lives. Chapter 5 looks at different theoretical perspectives offered by social science as explanations of quality of life. The contested nature of objective life quality and the subjective experience of older people are reflected within the different theories discussed. This issue dominates much of Chapter 6 in its review of the key issues in the assessment of quality of life and is one to which we return below.

Individual and societal perspectives

Taking the perspective of the individual recognizes that older people have agency, that is they are able to reflect on their social world and interact with it in order to influence the course and quality of their lives. The key idea here is the importance of the subjective experience in describing the nature of the social world. This subjectivist approach remains contested, however, because quality of life becomes a relative concept and, like relative poverty (Townsend 1970) and relative deprivation (Runciman 1966), is dismissed as not reflecting an objective reality (Hacking 1999). But we would question the existence of an objective reality when talking about quality of life. The fact that little correlation exists between an individual's subjective report of his or her world and an external objective description of the real world is highlighted by the lack of fit between reports of positive health status and the presence of chronic disease or the vision of happy smiling faces of some individuals living in abject absolute poverty. Like Townsend when defining relative poverty, or Runciman when explaining relative perceptions of social status, we would argue that an individual's own sense of the world may be more meaningful than an outsider's construction of objective reality. The societal perspective that imposes the dominant culture and its perspectives about the meaning, value and objective life quality risks establishing an account of quality of life that has little meaning to individuals within their own life world. This of course does not mean that consensus will not exist between people about some of the important features of people's lives. The studies of Bowling and Farquhar clearly show that consensus does exist but it would be wrong to typify a particular individual's quality of life on the basis of that individual's visible characteristics such as advanced age, disability or material circumstances. None of the domains illustrated in Hughes's model of quality of life shown in Table 1.1 (see Chapter 1) will be predictive for any given individual. The value in this kind of model is as a means of sensitizing us to the key issues in quality of life. It is an enormous epistemological, theoretical and methodological leap from understanding the individual worlds of older people to their predictive measurement. But such a perspective challenges the dominant positivist and post-positivist paradigms (Kuhn 1962) ways of investigating quality of life. In this final chapter we attempt to present an alternative approach to quality of life and older people. To do this we need to examine questions of ontology, epistemology, theory and method.

Quality of life and individual lived experience

Ontological questions are concerned with the nature of the knowable and the nature of reality. The fundamental question here is whether quality of life exists in the real world and whether it is something we can objectively describe and define. Is quality of life an objective (real) experience or is it a subjective experience mediated and described through the gaze of a parti-cular individual? Is quality of life something that we can predict and control? Natural and social scientists who argue that quality of life is something that we can describe and measure objectively, that it is an experience of the real world and therefore something that we can theoretically predict and control, are known as positivists. From a positivist perspective the lack of fit between objective measures of quality of life and reported subjective experiences can be explained by the quality of our measures or indicators of quality of life and the trustworthiness (or lack of it) of subjectivist accounts of quality of life. That objective definitions may be constructed by different individuals or social groups is not an explanation considered valid by positivists.

This position would appear to be rather naïve in the face of the paradox of objective and reported subjective experience. If quality of life remains an objective feature of everyday life that is driven by the natural world and subject to natural laws, its real nature is seen through the eyes of humans who interpret the real world and provide subjective accounts of quality of life. Social scientists who have adapted positivism in this way are known as post-positivists. That quality of life is an objective concept is central to their position. But there is recognition that objective definitions of quality of life are constructed differently by different members of society.

This is also the position taken by critical gerontology, bringing together the perspectives of feminism and post-Marxism, but the nature of objective reality is mediated by the values of individual actors as members of a complex stratified society. To some extent this may partly explain the paradox of objective experience and reported subjective experience of older people. The important question then becomes what values and whose values should govern the way we view quality of life? The choice of a particular value system tends to empower and enfranchise certain individuals and groups while disempowering and disenfranchising others. Defining quality of life therefore centrally becomes a political act and one that constructs and reconstructs the nature of quality of life.

We challenge the objective nature of quality of life accepted by the realist and critical realist ontologies of positivism, post-positivism and critical ger-ontology. Rather we view quality of life as a subjective lived experience that therefore exists in the form of multiple realities constructed and recon-structed by individual older people within the context of their different lives and life histories. Our argument takes the conventional composition of the constructionist account.

First, if quality of life is to have an objective reality like a tree or a house then it is essential that 'scientific' facts about the nature of quality of life are collected independently of any theoretical framework used to define quality of life. That such independence between the language of observation and theory is now recognized by philosophers of science to be impossible (Hesse 1980) means that objective reality only exists in the context of a mental framework or construct for thinking about it. Thus objective quality of life can only exist within theoretical frameworks that describe characteristics of quality of life in predetermined and fixed ways. It is unlikely that there exists consensus about the definitions presented.

Second, because of the philosophical problems of induction no theory can ever be fully tested. We are unable to say that 'the sun will always rise in the east', although our astronomical theories are reasonably robust on this point. But there will always be a number of plausible theories to explain quality of life. No unequivocal explanation will ever be possible. There will continue to be many constructions of quality of life and objective reality will therefore only be seen within the context of a given theoretical framework and through the gaze of individual theorists.

Third, we acknowledge that studying quality of life is not a value-free activity and that all facts are value-laden. So not only is quality of life seen through the gaze of individual theorists but also through the gaze of specific values multiplying the constructions available.

Thus ontologically there are always many interpretations of what is meant by quality of life and there exists no scientific process for establishing the ultimate objective reality. Rather we must accept that there is no alternative to relativism and the idea of multiple realities about quality of life. The meaning of quality of life lives in the individual's mind and seeking subjective accounts may be the only way to access them.

Epistemological questions are concerned with how we have knowledge of the external world and what the relationship is between the knower (inquirer) and the known (or knowable). A key question here is whether we (the inquirer) can perceive the real world of older people and in particular the lived experiences of individual older people. An assumption of positivists and post-positivists is that because we can define our own quality of life and what is important to our life quality we can do this for others. Critical theorists would argue that you can only understand the quality of life of the oppressed by being oppressed or by emancipating the oppressed to describe their own reality. So it is only women or people who are differently abled who can describe the lived experience of being a woman or being 'disabled'. A challenge here as Marx so cogently recognized is that it is only those who are oppressed and who have recognized their own oppression who will be in a position to present a realist view of their quality of life. From a constructionist perspective we would assume that multiple realities exist and that these realities are often relative to others. To understand life quality we would need to seek an understanding of what different aspects of life mean for the individual, the relative value of these different life aspects to the individual and the effect of context, particularly time and place. Such questions are complex and it is perhaps no surprise that inquirers revert to a positivist or post-positivist paradigm in which their own experiences and knowledge dictate the nature of the questions asked.

Investigating quality of life and individual lived experience

Methodological questions are concerned with how the inquirer should go about finding knowledge. These are important questions and reflect again the difference between objective and subjective definitions of quality of life. In Chapter 2 we presented the distinction made by Cornwell (1984) between public and private accounts and noted that in the context of a research interview the account provided by the study participant will depend on the nature of his or her relationship with the interviewer. This relationship will be influenced by a range of factors including the type and setting for the interview, the relative social status of the two participants in the interview and other contingencies in the life of the study participant. It is noteworthy that the setting of interviews, whether it is for research purposes, appraisal interviews in the workplace or interviews with police officers during criminal investigations, affects the way the interview is conducted and the kinds of accounts presented. Our experience of participating as subjects in such interviews suggests that we act differently when we are 'at home', in our own home or office, than we do in the more formal setting of a hospital or school, in the boss's office or in the local police station. The power of the interviewer increases when he or she dictates the setting and the kinds of questions to be asked.

The power of actors during interactions, of course, also relates to their relative position in the social order as reflected in their gender, age, ethnic status and 'social class', as well as their roles as professional or 'officials' in society. In our complex hierarchical society the accounts we provide are highly constrained by inequalities that exist within interactions. The power of actors during interactions is also affected by the type of power which is significant to the interaction. By power we mean the ways in which 'person A could cause person B to do something which was contrary to B's desire' (French and Raven 1968). A's dominant position during the interaction can be due to the power over rewards valued by B. Similarly A can control punishments. A's power can be legitimated by the organizational or societal context which may give him or her control over information, rights to access and rights to organize. In the research interview many of these different dimensions of power come into play such that the study participant becomes a 'vessel of data' (Holstein and Gubrium 1995) rather than an active participant.

The impact of life contingencies on controlled and directed data collection about quality of life extends the list of constraints that we have already identified for the research interview. Not least is the routine way that we respond to life events specifically and change more generally. Individual mood reflecting time and space and specific events can alter the way we respond in interviews, such that our public accounts change between interviews but have very little to do with a change in our quality of life. We reported these influences in Chapter 6 as part of the ongoing discourse about response shift in quality of life research.

Understanding quality of life and older people

In general, theoretical questions are concerned with how we explain past events and predict future events. The extent to which theory is used to predict future events will depend on the perspective adopted. Whereas positivists, post-positivists and critical theorists often invoke theory in prediction, constructionists only use theory as a means of explaining the past. Thus by taking a constructionist perspective we are arguing that we will be unable to provide a recipe for a good quality of life that will be suitable for all. Rather we can provide a coherent account of the diversity of lay explanations of life quality drawing on a range of theoretical perspectives from psychology, anthropology and sociology that examine both the individual and societal perspectives. From our theoretical account public policy could be addressed by government, statutory and voluntary organizations.

In Chapter 5 we lamented the poverty of theory in social gerontology and the hegemony of empiricism. In developing our theoretical account of quality of life we would wish to build on Jon Hendricks's credible attempts to build linkages between agency as reflected by individual subjectivity and structure, particularly dominant structural factors (Hendricks 2003). In summary the meaning that individuals give to the quality of their later life is probably determined by their life context: by the political, economic and cultural influences of the society in which they live; by individual lived experiences across the life course; by their current expectations, attitudes and values and by the context in which they reflectively provide this account. We have constructed a schematic framework that represents our theoretical account in Figure 7.1. In order to understand our account we expand on each element of the model in turn. A major challenge to our understanding of quality of life is the dynamic and interactive nature of most of the elements captured in the model. Thus in Chapter 2, for example, we introduced the idea of generational culture building on Mannheim's analysis of generational differences (Mannheim 1952). Each successive generation is experiencing increasing cultural, economic, political, social and technological change and this is reflected in differences in lifestyle, attitudes and expectations of ageing.

The influence of structure

The cultural, economic, political, social and technological context in which we all live is constantly changing and the rate of change continues to accelerate. Technological change is the key driver of economic change which in turn influences a much slower (even non-existent) change in our cultural, political and social institutions. Although critical gerontologists quite rightly have placed enormous weight on the significance of structural factors in explaining later life, the dynamic nature of cultural, political and social factors has been underplayed. It is only now with the postwar generation or 'baby boomers' generation reaching later years of the life course that cultural, economic, political and social change has been widely recognized.

As we saw in Chapter 5, feminist theory and political economy have made a substantive contribution to our understanding of the impact of structure on

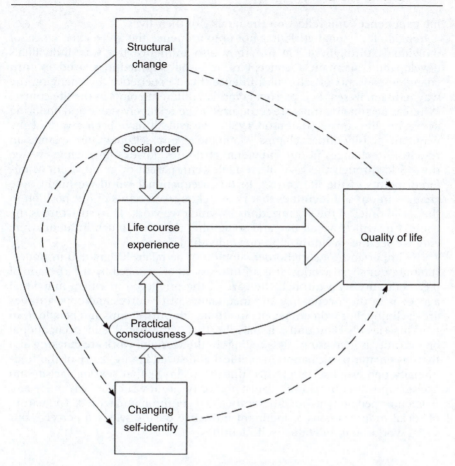

Figure 7.1   Schematic framework of the role of structure and ageing in the development and maintenance of quality of life through life-course experience

the lives of older people. Social order remains a key influence on life experience. Being born a white British male to parents with incomes and wealth within the top quintile of the income and wealth distribution endows the individual with substantial resources and opportunities. In contrast, being born a girl from a non-British ethnic minority group to parents earning below the minimum wage endows few resources and opportunities. It is often said that 'choosing the right parents' is a passport for a successful life. These individual attributes of gender, ethnicity, class and status at the beginning of life influence a person's subsequent lived experience along the whole life course. Although an individual's position in the social order clearly influences subsequent life course there is no indication that social position *per se* explains quality of life. Thus within the framework shown in Figure 7.1 social stratification and the changing nature and importance of it over time is seen as part of the broader social context in which individuals construct their own life experiences and reflect on the quality of their lives.

Individual personal attributes not only influence the 'lived experience' of individuals throughout life but they also influence the way individuals develop and maintain a concept of self and self-identities. And in turn changing concepts of self will influence 'lived experience' by changing the way individuals see their personal world at different points in the life course. Whereas personality traits are recognized to be relatively stable and enduring across the life course (Hampson 1988), we will all have been aware of the way our self-identities change. Sometimes our self-identities change in response to changes in our individual attributes, for example when we see the world through the gaze of an adolescent, parent or grandparent at different points of the life course. In our occupational world we might note changes in our self-identities that reflect changes in status or our position in the social order of the organizations in which we work. Thus structure is the context in which we all live and something that very much influences the way we see the world through our individual agency.

The importance of social order should not be taken for granted in understanding our social worlds. It is all too easy to be seduced by the rhetoric of postmodernity seen through the gaze of the privileged in which individual agency is in the ascendancy and inequalities of resources and opportunities are declining. For women, people in ethnic minority groups and people from working-class backgrounds, it may be that educational and occupational opportunity is increasing, glass ceilings in the world of work are cracking and there is greater participation in political and social life by many of the traditionally oppressed social groups. But the reality is that sexism, racism and ageism and discrimination against minority groups such as gay men and women or people who are differently abled continue unchecked. The nature of social order remains a dominant influence on the way we perceive our social worlds and individual self-identities.

Economic change and consumerism

With the collapse of state capitalism within the Soviet Union and Eastern Europe, the decline in the associated barriers to free trade and globalization of markets has increased the hegemony of capitalism. The importance of this economic order in our everyday lives is taken for granted and since the decline in the influence of Marxist and post-Marxist ideology is rarely critically evaluated. But the nature of the economic system is the dominant context in which we all live out our lives. The most tangible aspect of the economic order is not simply our increasing prosperity (and purchasing power) compared with previous generations, but the impact of consumerism in our everyday lives. We now all live in a consumer culture. It affects the way we live throughout the life course, influencing the structure of the labour market and the nature of employment opportunities, where we live and how we spend our leisure time and the kinds of commodities we desire and in some cases buy. In the framework of Figure 7.1 consumerism influences our personal attributes since we are all consumers in some shape or form.

But from our constructionist perspective consumerism also impacts on the way we each develop our self-identities and the way that others interact with us. Our personal identities are increasingly 'expressed, revised and represented through consumption' (Gilleard and Higgs 2000: 28). We saw in Chapter 4 how the development of the consumer culture had influenced the commodification of the body and of the ageing body. The clothes we wear, the cars we drive, the food we eat and the way we spend our leisure time are all part of the way we present ourselves in everyday life. Commodity brand names have become an important part of our self-image and affect the way others interact with us. Others will typify us according to our structural attributes (gender, age etc.), our consumer attributes and the way we present ourselves in everyday life. The impact of these typifications on our lived experience will vary according to the nature of the interaction, its social context and the degree to which our self-identity is accepted or challenged. The negative typifications often generated by the ageing body for example may lead to a decline in self-concept and a readjustment of self-identity. Of course, as we have seen in Chapter 4, such negative typifications of individuals tend to reflect the negative stereotypes of the social group and their cultural representation in society. The cultural representation of any social group therefore has a key role in describing an individual's personal attributes and influencing their lived experience across the life course.

Self-identity and quality of life

In our exposition of Figure 7.1 so far we have emphasized the broader influences of structure on 'lived experience' across the life course, particularly the role of the social and economic orders. We have argued that structure defines individual personal attributes that directly influence life-course experience. We have also argued that the context of structure and the definition of individual personal attributes has an important bearing upon the development and maintenance of self-identity by presenting self through the gaze and actions of others. However, the construction of self and self-identity is not the result of structure alone. As we saw in Chapter 5 the construction of self relies on a number of interactive elements in an individual's social and psychological experience. Importantly individuals act with agency. Agency embodies not only ideas from social action theory (Gerth and Mills 1948) and explanations of objective human action in terms of intention and rationality (Mead 1934). Agency is also about individual action, which is passionate and intuitive and distinctly subjective (Lash and Urry 1986). Individuals are able to think reflexively and formulate meaning from their individual experience. Reflexivity is the key cognitive process in individual action since it allows individuals to conceive themselves as a consequence of individual experience (Mead 1934).

How do we go about constructing our own self-identities? The key idea from constructionist theory is that our social world and the meanings we attach to it, including our own self-identities, are socially constituted (Berger and Luckmann 1966). During interactions with others, however brief, we jointly determine through negotiated meanings a shared definition of the situation. Achieving a successful interaction reinforces a shared under-standing of social reality. It is therefore by participation within social interactions that meaning is created. The creation of our own self-identity does not necessarily happen within the context of a single interaction. Rather self-identity develops through a number of interactions situated in a variety of contexts in time and space across the life course. An important feature of this process is that self-identity is not simply the creation of the individual's own imagination, although it plays an essential role, but the response and perception of others in the interaction. Thus over time personal identity is constructed and reconstructed in response to our experience of the social world in which we are participants. This process is a cognitive one and is captured by individual practical consciousness (Hendricks 1999) – the lens through which the individual gathers the whole range of sensory inputs within interactions and distils them into meaningful social experience. Thus practical consciousness is the link between the individual as a reflexive social actor and the subjectively created 'lived experience' at different points in time and space along the life course.

Practical consciousness has an important function in our framework for understanding quality of life in older people. It provides the vehicle for explaining the diversity of perspectives and meanings that older people report when describing their 'lived experiences'. But 'lived experience' is not determined by the individual alone or indeed by the range of structural factors identified above. Biology also plays a role with many key life events strongly associated with biological processes: physical and intellectual development, procreation and the whole ageing process. Of course, as we have already shown, we all provide a meaning to such natural biological processes. Serendipity or what Goffman (1961) described as contingencies also plays a role. Biology and individuals acting with agency all play a role in the birth of a child but it is serendipity that influences the timing of conception and birth. But our practical consciousness continues to make sense of each event however large or small that impacts on our own 'lived experience'.

'Lived experience' along the life course

A key principle of our framework for understanding quality of life (Figure 7.1) is the dynamic nature of the life course. As individuals we act out our lives in time (both chronological and historical) and space (both place and context). The differences in our life courses and life experiences are infinite as are the meanings we might give to different points on the life trajectory. Our 'lived experiences' will be the product of both structure and agency and it will be our lived experience that helps us understand our subjective assessment of our quality of lives. Thus it is the lived experience along the life course that mediates the effects of structure and agency and that would help us understand any given individual's subjective assessment of his or her quality of life at any particular point in time and space along the life course. Given the dynamic nature of the life course that reflects the changing context in which we all live, we would also expect quality of life to be dynamic with the possibility of subjective assessments of quality of life changing over time.

Rethinking quality of life

We started thinking about the issues in this book many years ago because we were unhappy with the interpretations of quality of life that many of our social science colleagues, biomedical scientists, policy makers and politicians were making. It became a difficult book to write because of the enormity of the literature on the subject and the need to provide a scholarly response to the dominance of positivism and post-positivism. In the process we have become far more sceptical about the use of the concept in applied social research and argue that we need to rethink quality of life research. We are not lone voices in this endeavour but the critics of quality of life are swamped by the armies of quality of life researchers pursuing their careers in one of the biggest social science industries of the late twentieth century. In this last section we wish to review our arguments and restate them in simple and quite stark terms.

Quality of life, we have argued, is a confusing and complex concept. It is used uncritically by many researchers and has taken on the mantle of the Holy Grail. Yet for older people it has common-sense meaning and one that could generate a range of lay theories and explanations. Although there are consistent accounts of what is important to older people in their everyday lives there remains a paradox about quality of life. Why is it that from an external observer's perspective some older people seem to live in undesirable social circumstances but are able to provide a positive subjective account of their quality of life? There are plausible explanations for this paradox within a constructionist perspective and the theoretical framework described in this chapter is one vehicle for examining such explanations. But if we follow this particular road there is little room for the battalions of positivist and post-positivists who declare the supremacy of so-called objective indicators of quality of life.

Our solution to this scholarly problem is to leave definitions of quality of life to individual actors functioning with agency in their own time and space. From this position we would suggest that the so-called objective indicators of quality of life remain simply social indicators and are assessed in their own right and not used as a proxy measure for the subjective experience called quality of life. This corresponds to our position on outcome measurement, which we have not articulated here. In summary we believe that the move towards generic measures of outcome in evaluation research devalues the contributions of individual factors. In outcome research quality of life is regularly used as the ultimate outcome. Its use may simplify statistical ana-lysis by providing a single dependent variable but it masks the contribution of specific aspects of quality of life that may be important in the context of the 'intervention'. Frequently in evaluation research this kind of outcome dis-criminates between experimental and non-experimental groups but we are often left with trying to understand what it is that the outcome represents in the life world of study participants.

We would propose that the way forward is to retain the term quality of life for everyday discourse where a shared understanding will emerge in the context of situated interactions between actors. In studying the lived experience of older people we should focus on their subjective accounts of well-being and keep separate within the analysis the objective social indicators such as health status, income and wealth, social support and social networks. This would not banish quality of life from our social research vocabulary, just from its use as a formalized psychometric concept. It would give us the freedom to use quality of life as a sensitizing concept and as a heuristic device for investigating the effects on older people of economic, social and technological change, public policy and everyday life events and experiences.

References

Abrams, M. (1973) Subjective social indicators, *Social Trends*, 4: 33–50.

Allen, I., Hogg, D. and Peace, S. (1992) *Elderly People: Choice, Participation and Satisfaction*. London: Policy Studies Institute.

Allen, I. and Perkins, E. (1995) *The Future of Family Care for Older People*. London: HMSO.

Alzheimer Scotland – Action on Dementia (2002) *You're Not Alone: Dementia Awareness in Scotland*. Edinburgh: Alzheimer Scotland – Action on Dementia.

Anderson, R. (1988) The quality of life of stroke patients and their carers. In Anderson, R. and Bury, M. (eds) *Living with Chronic Illness: The Experience of Patients and their Families*. London: Unwin Hyman.

Anderson, R. and Bury, M. (eds) (1988) *Living with Chronic Illlness: The Experience of Patients and their Families*. London: Unwin Hyman.

Andrews, F. M. and Withey, S. B. (1976) *Social Indicators of Well-Being: Americans' Perceptions of Life Quality*. New York: Plenum Press.

Andrews, M. (1999) The seductiveness of agelessness, *Ageing and Society*, 19: 301–18.

Aneshensel, C. S., Pearlin, L. I., Mullan, J. T., Zarit, S. H. and Whitlatch, C. J. (1995) *Profiles in Caregiving: The Unexpected Career*. San Diego, California: Academic Press.

Antonovsky, A. (1987) *Unraveling the Mystery of Health: How People Manage Stress and Stay Well*. San Francisco, California: Jossey-Bass.

Antonucci, T. C. and Akiyama, H. (1987) Social networks in adult life and a preliminary examination of the Convoy Model, *Journal of Gerontology*, 42 (5): 519–27.

Arber, S. and Ginn, J. (1991) *Gender and Later Life: A Sociological Analysis of Resources and Constraints*. London: Sage Publications.

Ariyoshi, S. (1987) *The Twilight Years* (published in Japanese in 1972), trans. Mildred Tahara. Tokyo: Kodansha International.

Atchley, R. C. (1989) A continuity theory of normal aging, *Gerontologist*, 29 (2): 183–90.

Atchley, R. C. (1998) Activity adaptations to the development of functional limitations and results for subjective well-being in later adulthood: a qualitative analysis of longitudinal panel data over a 16-year period, *Journal of Aging Studies*, 12 (1): 19–39.

Atkinson, A. B. (1995) *Incomes and the Welfare State*. Cambridge: Cambridge University Press.

Baltes, M. M. and Carstensen, L. L. (1996) The process of successful ageing, *Ageing and Society*, 16 (4): 397–422.

Baltes, P. B. and Baltes, M. M. (1980) Plasticity and variability in psychological aging: methodological and theoretical issues. In Gurski, G. E. (ed.) *Determining the Effects of Aging on the Central Nervous System*. Berlin: Schering AG.

Baltes, P. B. and Baltes, M. M. (1990a) Psychological perspectives on successful aging: the model of selective optimization with compensation. In Baltes, P. B. and Baltes, M. M. (eds) *Successful Aging: Perspectives from the Behavioral Sciences*. New York: Cambridge University Press.

Baltes, P. B. and Baltes, M. M. (eds) (1990b) *Successful Aging: Perspectives from the Behavioral Sciences*. Cambridge: Cambridge University Press.

Baltes, P. B., Dittmann-Kohli, F. and Dixon, R. A. (1984) New perspectives on the development of intelligence in adulthood: toward a dual-process conception and a model of selective optimization with compensation, *Life-Span Development and Behavior*, 6: 33–76.

Bamford, C. and Bruce, E. (2000) Defining the outcomes of community care: the perspectives of older people with dementia and their carers, *Ageing and Society*, 20: 543–70.

Bandura, A. (1981) Self-referent thought: a developmental analysis of self-efficacy. In Flavell, J. H. and Ross, L. (eds) *Social Cognitive Development: Frontiers and Possible Futures*. New York: Cambridge University Press.

Bauman, Z. (1988) Sociology and postmodernity, *Sociological Review*, 36: 790–813.

Bauman, Z. (1992) *Intimations of Postmodernity*. London: Routledge.

Becker, G. (1994) Age bias in stroke rehabilitation: effects on adult status, *Journal of Aging Studies*, 8 (3): 271–90.

Bengston, V. L. Burgess, E. O. and Parrott, T. M. (1997) Theory explanation, and a third generation of theoretical development in social gerontology, *Journal of Gerontology*, 52B(2), S72–S88.

Berger, P. and Luckmann, T. (1966) *The Social Construction of Reality*. Harmondsworth: Penguin.

Bernard, M. and Meade, K. (1993) A Third Age lifestyle for older women? In Bernard, M. and Meade, K. (eds) *Women Come of Age*. London: Edward Arnold.

Biggs, S. (1999) *The Mature Imagination: Dynamics of Identity in Midlife and Beyond*. Buckingham: Open University Press.

Blaikie, A. (1999) *Ageing and Popular Culture*. Cambridge: Cambridge University Press.

Blaikie, A. and Hepworth, M. (1997) Representations of old age in painting and photography. In Jamieson, A., Harper, S. and Victor, C. (eds) *Critical Approaches to Ageing and Later Life*. Buckingham: Open University Press.

Blakemore, K. and Boneham, M. (1994) *Age, Race and Ethnicity. A Comparative Approach*. Buckingham: Open University Press.

Blane, D., Wiggins, R., Higgs, P. and Hyde, M. (2002) Inequalities in quality of life in early old age, *Research Findings from the ESRC Growing Older Programme*, 9: 1–4.

Blaxter, M. (1990) *Health and Lifestyles*. London: Routledge.

Blaxter, M. and Paterson, E. (1982) *Mothers and Daughters: A Three Generational Study of Health Attitudes and Behaviour*. London: Heinemann Educational Books.

Blythe, R. (1979) *The View in Winter: Reflections on Old Age*. London: Allen Lane – Penguin Books Ltd.

Boleat, M. (1986) *Housing in Britain*. London: The Building Societies Association.

Bond, J. (1993a) Later life in a social context. In Day, P. R. (ed.) *Perspectives on Later Life: The Application of Research and Theory in Social Care*. London: Whiting & Birch.

Bond, J. (1993b) Living arrangements of elderly people. In Bond, J., Coleman, P. and Peace, S. (eds) *Ageing in Society. An Introduction to Social Gerontology*, 2nd edn. London: Sage Publications.

Bond, J. (1997) Health care reform in the UK: unrealistic or broken promises to older citizens, *Journal of Aging Studies*, 11 (3): 195–210.

Bond, J. (1999) Quality of life for people with dementia: approaches to the challenge of measurement, *Ageing and Society*, 19: 561–79.

Bond, J. (2000) The impact of staff factors on nursing-home residents [Editorial], *Aging and Mental Health*, 4 (1): 5–8.

Bond, J. (2001) Sociological perspectives. In Cantley, C. (ed.) *A Handbook of Dementia Care*. Buckingham: Open University Press.

Bond, J. and Bond, S. (1987) Development in the provision and evaluation of long-term care for dependent old people. In Fielding, P. (ed.) *Research in the Nursing Care of Elderly People*. London: Wiley.

Bond, J., Bond, S., Donaldson, C., Gregson, B. and Atkinson, A. (1989a) Evaluation of an innovation in the continuing care of very frail elderly people, *Ageing and Society*, 9: 347–81.

Bond, J., Briggs, R. and Coleman, P. (1993) The study of ageing. In Bond, J., Coleman, P. and Peace, S. (eds) *Ageing in Society. An Introduction to Social Gerontology*, 2nd edn. London: Sage Publications.

Bond, J. and Carstairs, V. (1982) *Services for the Elderly: A Survey of the Characteristics and Needs of a Population of 5,000 Old People*. Scottish Health Service Studies No. 42. Edinburgh: Scottish Home and Health Department.

Bond, J. and Corner, L. (2001) Researching dementia: are there unique methodological challenges for health services research?, *Ageing and Society*, 21 (1): 95–116.

Bond, J. and Corner, L. (2002) Being at risk of dementia: fears and anxieties of older adults, *Neurobiology of Aging*, 23 (1S): S542(Abstract).

Bond, J., Corner, L., Lilley, A. and Ellwood, C. (2002) Medicalisation of insight and caregivers' response to risk in dementia, *Dementia*, 1 (3): 313–28.

Bond, J., Gregson, B. A. and Atkinson, A. (1989b) Measurement of outcomes within a multicentred randomised controlled trial in the evaluation of the experimental NHS nursing homes, *Age and Ageing*, 18: 292–302.

Bond, S. and Bond, J. (1990) Outcomes of care within a multiple-case study in the evaluation of the experimental National Health Service Nursing Homes, *Age and Ageing*, 19: 11–18.

Booth, T. (1985) *Home Truths. Old People's Homes and the Outcome of Care*. Aldershot: Gower.

Booth, T., Bilson, A. and Fowell, I. (1990) Staff attitudes and caring practices in homes for the elderly, *British Journal of Social Work*, 20: 117–31.

Bowling, A. (1995a) *Measuring Disease*. Buckingham: Open University Press.

Bowling, A. (1995b) The most important things in life: comparisons between older and younger population age groups by gender: results from a national survey of the public's judgements, *International Journal of Health Sciences*, 6 (4): 169–75.

Bowling, A. (1995c) What things are important in people's lives? A survey of the public's judgements to inform scales of health related quality of life, *Social Science and Medicine*, 41 (10): 1447–62.

Bowling, A. (1996) *Measuring Health*, 2nd edn. Buckingham: Open University Press.

Bowling, A. and Browne, P. D. (1991) Social networks, health and emotional well-being among the oldest old in London, *Journal of Gerontology*, 46 (1) 520–32.

Bowling, A. and Farquhar, M. (1991) Life satisfaction and associations with social network and support variables in three samples of elderly people, *International Journal of Geriatric Psychiatry*, 6: 549–66.

Bowling, A., Gabriel, Z., Dykes, J. *et al.* (2003) Let's ask them: a national survey of definitions of quality of life and its enhancement among people aged 65 and over, *International Journal of Aging and Human Development*, 56 (4): 269–306.

Bowling, A., Grundy, E. and Farquhar, M. (1997) *Living Well into Old Age*. Social Care Research 95. York: Joseph Rowntree Foundation.

Bowling, A. and Windsor, J. (2001) Towards the good life: a population survey of dimensions of quality of life, *Journal of Happiness Studies*, 2: 55–81.

Brayne, C. and Ames, D. (1988) The epidemiology of mental disorder in old age. In Gearing, B., Johnson, M. L. and Heller, T. (eds) *Mental Health Problems in Old Age*. Chichester: Wiley.

Bridgwood, A. (2000) *People Aged 65 and Over: Results of an Independent Study Carried Out on Behalf of the Department of Health as Part of the 1998 General Household Survey*. London: Office for National Statistics.

Brown, G. W. and Harris, T. (1978) *Social Origins of Depression. A Study of Psychiatric Disorder in Women*. London: Tavistock Publications.

Brunswick, E. (1956) *Perception and the Representative Design of Psychological Experiments*. Berkeley, California: University California Press.

Burgess, E. W. (1954) Social relations, activities, and personal adjustment, *American Journal of Sociology*, 59 (4): 352–60.

Burholt, V. and Wenger, G. C. (1998) Differences over time in older people's relationships with children and siblings, *Ageing and Society*, 18: 537–62.

Bury, M. (1982) Chronic illness as biographical disruption, *Sociology of Health and Illness*, 4 (2): 167–82.

Bury, M. (1988) Meanings at risk: the experience of arthritis. In Anderson, R. and Bury, M. (eds) *Living with Chronic Illness. The Experience of Patients and Their Families*. London: Unwin Hyman.

Bury, M. (1991) The sociology of chronic illness: a review of research and prospects, *Sociology of Health and Illness*, 13 (4): 451–68.

Bury, M. (1995) Ageing, gender and sociological theory. In Arber, S. and Ginn, J. (eds) *Connecting Gender and Ageing: A Sociological Approach*. Buckingham and Philadelphia, Pennsylvania: Open University Press.

Bury, M. and Holme, A. (1990) Quality of life and social support in the very old, *Journal of Aging Studies*, 4 (4): 345–57.

Butler, R. N. (1987) Ageism. In *The Encyclopedia of Aging*. New York: Springer.

Bytheway, B. (1995) *Rethinking Ageing: Ageism*. Buckingham: Open University Press.

Campbell, A. (1981) *The Sense of Well-being in America: Recent Patterns and Trends*. New York: McGraw-Hill Book Company.

Carley, M. (1981) *Social Measurement and Social Indicators: Issues of Policy and Theory*. London: Allen & Unwin.

Carr, A. J., Higginson, I. J. and Robinson, P. G. (eds) (2003) *Quality of Life*. London: BMJ Books.

Carrigan, M. and Szmigin, I. (2000) Advertising in an ageing society, *Ageing and Society*, 20 (2): 217–33.

Centre for Policy on Ageing (1984) *Home Life: A Code of Practice for Residential Care*. London: Centre for Policy on Ageing.

Challiner, Y., Julious, S., Watson, R. and Philp, I. (1996) Quality of care, quality of life and the relationship between them in long-term care institutions for the elderly, *International Journal of Geriatric Psychiatry*, 11: 883–8.

Charmaz, K. (1983) Loss of self: a fundamental form of suffering in the chronically ill, *Sociology of Health and Illness*, 5 (2): 168–95.

Charmaz, K. (1987) Struggling for a self. In Roth, J. A. and Conrad, P. (eds) *Identity Levels of the Chronically Ill*, London and Greenwich, Connecticut: JAI Press Inc.

Charmaz, K. (2000) Experiencing chronic illness. In Albrecht, G. L., Fitzpatrick, R. and Scrimshaw, S. C. (eds) *Handbook of Social Studies in Health and Medicine*. London: Sage Publications.

Chipperfield, J. G. and Havens, B. (2001) Gender differences in the relationship between marital status transitions and life satisfaction in later life, *Journal of Gerontology*, 56B (3): 176–86.

Coleman, P. (1986) Adjustment to later life. In Bond, J. and Coleman, P. (eds) *Ageing in Society. An Introduction to Social Gerontology*. London: Sage Publications.

Coleman, P. G. (1984) Assessing self-esteem and its sources in elderly people, *Ageing and Society*, 4: 117–35.

Coleman, P. G., McKiernan, F., Mills, M. and Speck, P. (2002) Spiritual belief and quality of life: the experience of older bereaved spouses, *Quality in Ageing – Policy, practice and research*, 3 (1): 20–6.

Comfort, A. (1977) *A Good Age*. London: Mitchell Beazley.

Cooley, C. H. (1902) *Human Nature and the Social Order*. New York: Charles Scribner.

Corbin, J. M. and Strauss, A. (1988) *Unending Work and Care: Managing Chronic Illness at Home*. London and San Francisco, California: Jossey-Bass.

Corner, L. (1999) Developing approaches to person-centred outcome measures for older people in rehabilitation settings. Unpublished PhD thesis, University of Newcastle upon Tyne.

Corner, L. and Bond, J. (2004) Being at risk of dementia: fears and anxieties of older adults, *Journal of Aging Studies*, 18 (2): 143–155.

Cornwell, J. (1984) *Hard-earned Lives: Accounts of Health and Illness from East London*. London: Tavistock.

Cumming, E. and Henry, W. E. (1961) *Growing Old: The Process of Disengagement*. New York: Basic Books.

Cutler, S. J. and Hodgson, L. G. (1996) Anticipatory dementia: a link between memory appraisals and concerns about developing Alzheimer's disease, *Gerontologist*, 36 (5): 657–64.

Dale, A., Evandrou, M. and Arber, S. (1987) The household structure of the elderly population in Britain, *Ageing and Society*, 7: 37–56.

Dant, T. (1988) Dependency and old age: theoretical accounts and practical understandings, *Ageing and Society*, 8: 171–88.

Davis, I., Leigh, S., Parry, S., Kent, C. and Nicholls, M. (eds) (2003) *The Pensioners' Incomes Series 2001/2*. London: Department for Work and Pensions.

DHSS (Department of Health and Social Security) (1983a) *Elderly People in the Community: Their Service Needs*. London: HMSO.

DHSS (1983b) *The Experimental National Health Service Nursing Homes for Elderly People. An Outline*. London: DHSS.

Dilnot, A., Disney, R., Johnson, P. and Whitehouse, E. (1994) *Pensions Policy in the UK. An Economic Analysis*. London: Institute for Fiscal Studies.

DoH (Department of Health) (2001) *National Service Framework for Older People*. London: NHS Executive.

Durkheim, E. (1964) *The Division of Labour in Society*. New York: Free Press.

Estes, C. L. (1979) *The Aging Enterprise. A Critical Examination of Social Policies and Services for the Aged*. San Francisco, California: Jossey-Bass.

Estes, C. L., Alford, R. R., Binney, E. A. *et al.* (2001) *Social Policy and Aging: A Critical Perspective*. Thousand Oaks, California: Sage.

Estes, C. L. and Binney, E. (1989) The biomedicalisation of aging: dangers and dilemmas, *Gerontologist*, 29 (5): 587–96.

Estes, C. L., Swan, J. H. and Gerard, L. E. (1982) Dominant and competing paradigms in gerontology: towards a political economy of ageing, *Ageing and Society*, 2: 151–64.

Eurostat (1996) *Digest of Statistics on Social Protection in Europe. Old Age and Survivors: An Update.* Luxembourg: Office for Official Publications of the European Communities.

Falkingham, J. and Victor, C. (1991) The myth of the Woopie? Incomes, the elderly and targeting welfare, *Ageing and Society*, 11: 471–93.

Farquhar, M. (1994) Quality of life in older people. In Fitzpatrick, R. (ed.) *Advances in Medical Sociology.* Greenwich, Connecticut: JAI Press Inc.

Farquhar, M. (1995) Elderly people's definitions of quality of life, *Social Science and Medicine*, 41 (10): 1439–46.

Featherman, D. L., Smith, J. and Peterson, J. G. (1990) Successful aging in a post-retired society. In Baltes, P. B. and Baltes, M. M. (eds) *Successful Aging: Perspectives from the Behavioral Sciences.* New York: Cambridge University Press.

Featherstone, M. (1991) The body in consumer culture. In Featherstone, M., Hepworth, M. and Turner, B. S. (eds) *The Body: Social Process and Cultural Theory.* London: Sage Publications.

Featherstone, M. and Hepworth, M. (1989) Ageing and old age: reflections on the postmodern life course. In Bytheway, B., Keil, T., Allatt, P. and Bryman, A. (eds) *Becoming and Being Old: Sociological Approaches to Later Life.* London: Sage Publications.

Featherstone, M. and Hepworth, M. (1991) The mask of ageing and postmodern life course. In Featherstone, M., Hepworth, M. and Turner, B. S. (eds) *The Body: Social Process and Cultural Theory.* London: Sage Publications.

Featherstone, M. and Hepworth, M. (1993) Images of ageing. In Bond, J., Coleman, P. and Peace, S. (eds) *Ageing in Society. An Introduction to Social Gerontology*, 2nd edn. London: Sage Publications.

Featherstone, M. and Hepworth, M. (1995) Images of positive aging: a case study of *Retirement Choice* magazine. In Featherstone, M. and Warwick, A. (eds) *Images of Aging: Cultural Representations of Later Life.* London: Routledge.

Featherstone, M. and Wernick, A. (eds) (1995) *Images of Aging: Cultural Representations of Later Life.* London and New York: Routledge.

Fennell, G., Phillipson, C. and Evers, H. (1988) *The Sociology of Old Age.* Milton Keynes: Open University Press.

Fernández-Ballesteros, R., Zamarrón, M. D. and Ruíz, M. A. (2001) The contribution of socio-demographic and psychosocial factors to life satisfaction, *Ageing and Society*, 21 (1): 25–43.

Finch, J. and Mason, J. (1993) *Negotiating Family Responsibilities.* London: Routledge.

Fisher, B. J. (1992) Successful aging and life satisfaction: a pilot study for conceptual clarification, *Journal of Aging Studies*, 6 (2): 191–202.

Fitzpatrick, R., Davey, C., Buxton, M. J. and Jones, D. R. (1998) Patient-assessed outcome measures. In Black, N., Brazier, J., Fitzpatrick, R. and Reeves, B. (eds) *Health Services Research Methods. A Guide to Best Practice.* London: BMJ Books.

Foresight Ageing Population Panel (2000) *The Age Shift – Priorities for Action.* London: Department of Trade and Industry.

Fox, N. J. (1993) *Postmodernism, Sociology and Health.* Buckingham: Open University Press.

Freidson, E. (1975) *Profession of Medicine. A Study of the Sociology of Applied Knowledge.* New York: Dodd, Mead & Co.

French, J. R. P. and Raven, B. (1968) The Bases of Social Power. In Cartwright, D. and Zander, A. (eds) *Group Dynamics. Research and Theory*, 3rd edn. New York: Harper & Row.

Fries, J. F. and Crapo, L. M. (1981) *Vitality and Aging. Implications of the Rectangular Curve.* San Francisco, California: W. H. Freeman.

Fry, P. S. (2000) Whose quality of life is it anyway? Why not ask seniors to tell us about it?, *International Journal of Aging and Human Development*, 50 (4): 361–83.

Galbraith, J. K. (1962) *The Affluent Society*. Victoria, Australia: Pelican Books.

Gecas, V. and Burke, P. J. (1995) Self and identity. In Cook, K. S., Fine, G. A. and House, J. S. (eds) *Sociological Perspectives on Social Psychology*. Boston, Massachusetts: Allyn and Bacon.

George, L. K. (1979) The happiness syndrome: methodological and substantive issues in the study of social-psychological well-being in adulthood, *Gerontologist*, 19 (2): 210–15.

George, L. K. and Bearon, L. B. (1980) *Quality of Life in Older Persons. Meaning and Measurement*. New York: Human Sciences Press.

George, L. K., Larson, D. B., Koenig, H. G. and McCullough, M. E. (2000) Spirituality and health: what we know, what we need to know, *Journal of Social and Clinical Psychology*, 19: 102–16.

Gergen, K. J. and Davis, K. E. (eds) (1985) *The Social Construction of the Person*. New York: Springer Verlag.

Gerth, H. H. and Mills, C. W. (1948) *From Max Weber: Essays in Sociology*. London: Routledge and Kegan Paul.

Giddens, A. (1976) *New Rules of Sociological Method: A Positive Critique of Interpretative Sociologies*. London: Hutchinson.

Giddens, A. (1991) *Modernity and Self-identity: Self and Society in the Late Modern Age*. Cambridge: Polity Press.

Giddens, A. and Birdsall, K. (2001) *Sociology*, 4th edn. Cambridge: Polity Press.

Gieryn, T. F. (1983) Boundary work and the demarcation of science from non-science: strains and interests in the professional ideologies of scientists, *American Sociological Review*, 48 (6): 781–95.

Giles, H. and Coupland, N. (1991) *Language: Contexts and Consequences*. Pacific Grove, California: Brooks/Cole Publishing Company.

Gilleard, C. and Higgs, P. (2000) *Cultures of Ageing: Self, Citizen and the Body*. Harlow: Prentice-Hall.

Gilleard, C. and Higgs, P. (2002) Concept Forum. The third age: class, cohort or generation?, *Ageing and Society*, 22 (3): 369–82.

Goddard, E. and Savage, D. (1994) *1991 General Household Survey: People Aged 65 and Over*. Series GHS no. 22, London: OPCS.

Goffman, E. (1961) *Asylum: Essays on the Social Situation of Mental Patients and Other Inmates*. New York: Anchor Books.

Goffman, E. (1968) *Stigma: Notes on the Management of Spoiled Identity*. Harmondsworth: Penguin Books.

Goffman, E. (1971) *The Presentation of Self in Everyday Life*. Harmondsworth: Penguin Books.

Goldberg, D. and Williams, P. (1988) *A User's Guide to the General Health Questionnaire*. Windsor: NFER-Nelson Publishing Company Ltd.

Graney, M. J. (1975) Happiness and social participation in aging, *Journal of Gerontology*, 30 (6): 701–6.

Gubrium, J. F. (1986) *Oldtimers and Alzheimer's: The Descriptive Organization of Senility*. London: Jai Press Inc.

Gubrium, J. F. (1987) Structuring and destructuring the course of illness: the Alzheimer's disease experience, *Sociology of Health and Illness*, 9: 1–24.

Gubrium, J. F. and Lynott, R. J. (1983) Re-thinking life satisfaction, *Human Organization*, 42: 30–8.

Gurland, B. and Katz, S. (1992) The outcomes of psychiatric disorder in the elderly: relevance to quality of life. In Birren, J. E., Sloane, R. B. and Cohen, G. D. (eds) *Handbook of Mental Health and Aging*. San Diego, California: Academic Press.

Hacking, I. (1999) *The Social Construction of What?* Cambridge, Massachusetts: Harvard University Press.

Hall, J. (1976) Subjective measures of quality of life in Britain: 1971 to 1975. In: *Social Trends*, No. 7. Abington: Burgess and Son.

Hampson, S. E. (1988) *The Construction of Personality: An Introduction*, 2nd edn. London and New York: Routledge.

Hancock, R. (1998) Housing wealth, income and financial wealth of older people in Britain, *Ageing and Society*, 18: 5–33.

Havighurst, R. J. (1963) Successful ageing. In Williams, R. H., Tibbitts, C. and Donahue, W. (eds), *Processes of Ageing*. New York: Atherton.

Hazan, H. (1980) *The Limbo People: A Study of the Constitution of the Time Universe Among the Aged*. London: Routledge and Kegan Paul.

Hazan, H. (1994) *Old Age: Constructions and Deconstructions*. Cambridge: Cambridge University Press.

Heim, A. (1990) *Where Did I Put My Spectacles?* Cambridge: Albrough Press.

Hendricks, J. (1999) Practical consciousness, social class, and self-concept: a view from sociology. In Ryff, C. D. and Marshall, V. W. (eds) *The Self and Society in Aging Processes*. New York: Springer Publishing Co.

Hendricks, J. (2003) Structure and identity – mind the gap: toward a personal resource model of successful ageing. In Biggs, S., Lowenstein, A. and Hendricks, J. (eds). *The Need for Theory: Critical Approaches to Social Gerontology*. Amityville, NY: Baywood Publishing Company, Inc.

Henwood, M. (1990) No sense of urgency: age discrimination in health care. In McEwen, E. (ed.) *The Unrecognised Discrimination*. London: Age Concern England.

Hepworth, M. (2000) *Stories of Ageing*. Buckingham and Philadelphia, Pennsylvania: Open University Press.

Herzlich, C. (1973) *Health and Illness*. London: Academic Press.

Herzlich, C. and Pierret, J. (1987) *Illness and Self in Society*. Baltimore, Maryland: Johns Hopkins University Press.

Hesse, M. (1980) *Revolutions and Reconstructions in the Philosophy of Science*. Brighton: The Harvester Press.

Hislop, L. J., Wyatt, J. P., McNaughton, G. W. *et al.* (1995) The West of Scotland Accident and Emergency Trainees Research Group. Urban hypothermia in the west of Scotland, *British Medical Journal*, 311 (7007): 725.

Hockey, J. and James, A. (1993) *Growing Up and Growing Old. Ageing and Dependency in the Life Course*. London: Sage Publications.

Hodgson, L. G. and Cutler, S. J. (1997) Anticipatory dementia and well-being, *American Journal of Alzheimer's Disease*, (March/April): 62–6.

Hogan, D. B. and McKeith, I. G. (2001) Of MCI and dementia: improving diagnosis and treatment, *Neurology*, 56: 1131–2.

Holstein, J. A. and Gubrium, J. F. (1995) *The Active Interview*. Thousand Oaks, California: Sage Publications.

Holstein, M. (2000) Aging, culture, and the framing of Alzheimer disease. In Whitehouse, P. J., Maurer, K. and Ballenger, J. F. (eds) *Concepts of Alzheimer Disease: Biological, Clinical, and Cultural Perspectives*. Baltimore, Maryland and London: Johns Hopkins University Press.

Horgas, A. L., Wilms, H.-U. and Baltes, M. M. (1998) Daily life in very old age: everyday activities as expression of successful living, *Gerontologist*, 38 (5): 556–68.

Hughes, B. (1990) Quality of life. In Peace, S. M. (ed.) *Researching Social Gerontology*. London: Sage Publications.

Hughes, B. and Wilkin, D. (1987) Physical care and quality of life in residential homes, *Ageing and Society*, 7: 399–425.

Hunt, A. (1978a) *The Elderly at Home: A Study of People Aged 65 and Over Living in the Community in England in 1976*. London: HMSO.

Hunt, A. (1978b) The elderly: age differences in the quality of life, *Population Trends*, 11: 10–15.

Husband, H. J. (2000) Diagnostic disclosure in dementia: an opportunity for intervention?, *International Journal of Geriatric Psychiatry*, 15: 544–7.

Idler, E. L. and Benyamini, Y. (1997) Self-rated health and mortality: a review of twenty-seven community studies, *Journal of Health and Social Behaviour*, 38: 21–37.

Itzin, C. (1986) Ageism awareness training: a model for group work. In Phillipson, C., Bernard, M. and Strang, P. (eds) *Dependency and Interdependency in Old Age: Theoretical Perspectives and Policy Alternatives*. London: Croom Helm.

Jerrome, D. (1984) Good company: the sociological implications of friendship, *Sociological Review*, 32: 696–718.

Jerrome, D. (1993) Intimate relationships. In Bond, J., Coleman, P. and Peace, S. (eds) *Ageing in Society. An Introduction to Social Gerontology*, 2nd edn. London: Sage Publications.

Jerrome, D. and Wenger, G. C. (1999) Stability and change in late-life friendships, *Ageing and Society*, 19: 661–76.

Johnson, J. and Bytheway, B. (1993) Ageism: concept and definition. In Johnson, J. and Slater, R. (eds) *Ageing and Later Life*. London: Sage Publications.

Johnson, P. and Falkingham, J. (1992) *Ageing and Economic Welfare*. London: Sage Publications.

Johnson, P. and Stears, G. (1997) *Why are Older Pensioners Poorer?* London: Institute for Fiscal Studies.

Joint Taskforce on Older People (2000) *Healthcare and Ageing Population Panels*, London: Department of Trade and Industry.

Jones, D. A., Victor, C. R. and Vetter, N. J. (1985) The problem of loneliness in the elderly in the community: characteristics of those who are lonely and the factors related to loneliness, *Journal of the Royal College of General Practitioners*, 35: 136–9.

Jorm, A. F., Korten, A. E. and Henderson, A. S. (1987) The prevalence of dementia: a quantitative integration of the literature, *Acta Psychiatrica Scandinavia*, 76: 465–79.

Katzman, R. and Bick, K. L. (2000) The rediscovery of Alzheimer disease during the 1960s and 1970s. In Whitehouse, P. J., Maurer, K. and Ballenger, J. F. (eds) *Concepts of Alzheimer Disease: Biological, Clinical, and Cultural Perspectives*. Baltimore, Maryland and London: Johns Hopkins University Press.

Keatinge, W. R. (1986) Seasonal mortality among elderly people with unrestricted home heating, *British Medical Journal*, 293: 732–3.

Kelly, G. A. (1955) *The Psychology of Personal Constructs*. New York: W.W. Norton & Company.

Kennedy, C. A., King, J. A. and Muraco, W. A. (1991) The relative strength of health as a predictor of life satisfaction, *International Social Science Review*, 97–102.

Kirkwood, T. (1999) *Time of our Lives: The Science of Human Ageing*. London: Weidenfeld and Nicolson.

Koenig, H. G. (1993) Religion and aging, *Reviews in Clinical Gerontology*, 3: 195–203.

Koenig, H. G. (1995) Religion and health in later life. In Kimble, M. A., McFadden, S. H., Ellor, J. W. and Seeber, J. J. (eds) *Aging, Spirituality and Religion*. Minneapolis, Minnesota: Fortress Press.

Kuhn, T. S. (1962) *The Structure of Scientific Revolutions*. Chicago, Illinois: Chicago University Press.

Kutner, B., Fanshel, D., Togo, A. M. and Langner, T. S. (1956) *Five Hundred Over Sixty: A Community Survey on Aging*. New York: Russell Sage Foundation.

Laczko, F. and Phillipson, C. (1990) Defending the right to work: age discrimination in employment. In McEwen, E. (ed.) *Age: The Unrecognised Discrimination*. London: Age Concern.

Laczko, F. and Phillipson, C. (1991) *Changing Work and Retirement*. Milton Keynes: Open University Press.

Larrieu, S., Letenneur, L., Orgogozo, J. M. *et al.* (2002) Incidence and outcome of mild cognitive impairment in a population-based prospective cohort, *Neurology*, 59: 1594–9.

Larson, R. (1978) Thirty years of research on the subjective well-being of older Americans, *Journal of Gerontology*, 33 (1): 109–25.

Lash, S. and Urry, J. (1986) Dissolution of the social? In Wardell, M. L. and Turner, S. P. (eds) *Sociological Theory in Transition*. London: Sage Publications.

Laslett, P. (1977) The history of ageing and the aged. In Laslett, P., *Family Life and Illicit Love in Earlier Generations*. Cambridge: Cambridge University Press.

Laslett, P. (1987) The emergence of the third age, *Ageing and Society*, 7: 133–60.

Laslett, P. (1996) *A Fresh Map of Life: The Emergence of the Third Age*, 2nd edn. London: Weidenfeld and Nicolson.

Lemon, B. W., Bengtson, V. L. and Peterson, J. A. (1972) An exploration of the activity theory of aging: activity types and life satisfaction among in-movers to a retirement community, *Journal of Gerontology*, 27 (4): 511–23.

Leplege, A. and Hunt, S. (1997) The problem of quality of life in medicine, *Journal of the American Medical Association*, 278 (1): 47–50.

Levinson, D. J. (1990) A theory of life structure development in adulthood. In Alexander, C. N. and Langer, E. J. (eds) *Higher Stages of Human Development: Perspectives on Adult Growth*. New York: Oxford University Press.

Lowenthal, M. F. and Haven, C. (1968) Interaction and adaptation: intimacy as a critical variable, *American Sociological Review*, 33 (1): 20–30.

McCall, S. (1975) Quality of life, *Social Indicators Research*, 2: 229–48.

McColl, E., Christiansen, T. and Konig-Zahn, C. (1997) Making the right choice of outcome measure. In Hutchinson, A., Bentzen, N., Konig-Zahn, C. *et al.* (eds) *Cross Cultural Health Outcome Assessment*, Groningen: University of Groningen.

McConaghy, M., Foster, K., Thomas, M., Grove, J. and Oliver, R. (2000) *Housing in England 1998/99*. London: The Stationery Office.

McCormick, A., Fleming, D. and Charlton, J. (1995) *Morbidity Statistics from General Practice: Fourth National Study*. London: OPCS.

Macdonald, B. and Rich, C. (1984) *Look Me In the Eye: Old Women, Aging and Ageism*. San Francisco, California: Spinsters, Ink.

McDowell, I. and Newell, C. (1987) *Measuring Health: A Guide to Rating Scales and Questionnaires*. New York: Oxford University Press.

McFadden, S. H. (1999) Religion, personality, and aging: a life span perspective, *Journal of Personality*, 67: 1081–104.

Maddox, G. L. (1963) Activity and morale: a longitudinal study of selected elderly subjects, *Social Forces*, 42: 195–204.

Maddox, G. L. (1969) Themes and issues in sociological theories of human aging. In *8th International Congress of Gerontology: Proceedings – Volume 1*. Washington, DC: International Association of Gerontology.

Mannheim, K. (1952) The problem of generations. In Kecskemeti, P. (ed.) *Essays on the Sociology of Knowledge*. London: Routledge and Kegan Paul.

Markson, E. W. and Taylor, C. A. (2000) The mirror has two faces, *Ageing and Society*, 20 (2): 137–60.

Marris, P. (1958) *Widows and their Families*. London: Routledge and Kegan Paul.

Marris, P. (1986) *Loss and Change*, 2nd edn. London: Routledge and Kegan Paul.

Mead, G. H. (1934) *Mind, Self and Society*. Chicago, Illinois: University of Chicago Press.

Medical Research Council (1994) *The Health of the UK's Elderly People*. London: Medical Research Council.

Minkler, M. and Estes, C. L. (eds) (1999) *Critical Gerontology: Perspectives from Political and Moral Economy*. Amityville, New York: Baywood.

MRC CFAS (1998) Cognitive function and dementia in six areas of England and Wales: the distribution of MMSE and prevalence of GMS organicity level in the MRC CFA study, *Psychological Medicine*, 28: 319–35.

MRC CFAS (Medical Research Council Cognitive Function and Ageing Study) and RIS MRC CFAS (Resource Implications Study) (1999) Profile of disability in elderly people: estimates from a longitudinal population study, *British Medical Journal*, 318: 1108–11.

MRC CFAS (2001) Health and ill-health in the older population in England and Wales, *Age and Ageing*, 30: 53–62.

Mroczek, D. K. and Kolarz, M. (1998) The effect of age on positive and negative affect: a developmental perspective on happiness, *Journal of Personality and Social Psychology*, 75 (5): 1333–49.

Murphy, E., Dingwall, R., Greatbatch, D., Parker, S. and Watson, P. (1998) Qualitative research methods in health technology assessment: a review of the literature, *Health Technology Assessment*, 2(16).

Neisser, U. and Jopling, D. A. (eds) (1997) *The Conceptual Self in Context: Culture Experience Self-understanding*. Cambridge: Cambridge University Press.

Nettleton, S. (1995) *The Sociology of Health and Illness*. Cambridge: Polity Press.

Neugarten, B. L., Havighurst, R. J. and Tobin, S. S. (1961) The measurement of life satisfaction, *Journal of Gerontology*, 16: 134–43.

Neuropathology Group of the Medical Research Council Cognitive Function and Ageing Study (MRC CFAS) (2001) Pathological correlates of late-onset dementia in a multicentre, community-based population in England and Wales, *The Lancet*, 357 (9251): 169–75.

O'Boyle, C. A., McGee, H., Hickey, A., O'Malley, K. and Joyce, C. R. B. (1989) Reliability and validity of judgement analysis as a method for assessing quality of life, *British Journal of Clinical Pharmacology*, 27: 155.

O'Boyle, C. A., McGee, H. and Joyce, C. R. B. (1994) Quality of life: assessing the individual. In Fitzpatrick, R. (ed.) *Advances in Medical Sociology*. Greenwich, Connecticut: JAI Press.

Okun, M. A., Stock, W. A., Haring, M. J. and Witter, R. A. (1984) Health and subjective wellbeing: a meta-analysis, *International Journal of Aging and Human Development*, 19: 111–32.

ONS (Office for National Statistics) (2003) *Census 2001: National Report for England and Wales*. London: The Stationery Office.

OPCS (1982) *General Household Survey 1980*. London: HMSO.

OPCS/GRO(S) (1993) *1991 Census. Persons aged 60 and over, Great Britain*. London: HMSO.

Pacolet, J., Bouten, R., Lanoye, H. and Versieck, K. (2000) *Social Protection for Dependency in Old Age: A Study of the Fifteen EU Member States and Norway*. Aldershot: Ashgate.

Palmore, E. and Luikart, C. (1972) Health and social factors related to life satisfaction, *Journal of Health and Social Behavior*, 13: 68–80.

Phillipson, C. (1982) *Capitalism and the Construction of Old Age*. London: Macmillan.

Phillipson, C. (1998) *Reconstructing Old Age: New Agendas in Social Theory and Practice*. London: Sage Publications.

Phillipson, C., Bernard, M., Phillips, J. and Ogg, J. (2001) *The Family and Community Life of Older People: Social Networks and Social Support in Three Urban Areas*. London: Routledge.

Pinder, R. (1988) Striking balances: living with Parkinson's disease. In Anderson, R. and Bury, M. (eds) *Living with Chronic Illness. The Experience of Patients and Their Families*. London: Unwin Hyman Ltd.

Puner, M. (1974) *To the Good Long Life: What We Know About Growing Old*. London: Macmillan Press.

Qureshi, H. (1994) Impact on families: young adults with learning disability who show challenging behaviour. In Kiernan, C. (ed.) *Research to Practice? Implications of Research on the Challenging Behaviour of People with Learning Disability*. Clevedon: British Institute of Learning Disability.

Qureshi, H., Patmore, C., Nicholas, E. and Bamford, C. (1998) *Overview: Outcomes of Social Care for Older People and Carers*. Outcomes in Community Care Practice, No. 5. York: Social Policy Research Unit, University of York.

Qureshi, H. and Walker, A. (1989) *The Caring Relationship. Elderly People and their Families*. London: Macmillan.

Rabbitt, P. M. A. (1992) Memory. In Evans, J. G. and Williams, F. T. (eds) *Oxford Handbook of Geriatric Medicine*. London: Oxford University Press.

Radley, A. and Green, R. (1987) Illness as adjustment: a methodology and conceptual framework, *Sociology of Health and Illness*, 9: 179–207.

Rapley, M. (2003) *Quality of Life Research: A Critical Introduction*. London: Sage Publications.

Ray, R. E. (1996) A postmodern perspective on feminist gerontology, *Gerontologist*, 36 (5): 674–80.

Reichard, S., Livson, F. and Peterson, P. G. (1962) *Aging and Personality: A Study of Eighty-seven Older Men*. New York: John Wiley & Sons.

Riley, B. B., Perna, R., Tate, D. G. *et al.* (1998) Types of spiritual well-being among persons with chronic illness: their relation to various forms of quality of life, *Archives of Physical Medicine and Rehabilitation*, 79: 258–64.

Riley, M. W., Johnson, M. and Foner, A. (1972) A Sociology of Age Stratification. In Riley, M. W., Foner, A., Moore, M. E., Hers, B. and Roth, B. K. (eds) *Ageing and Society*, Vol. 3. New York: Russell Sage.

RIS MRC CFAS Resource Implications Study Group of the Medical Research Council Cognitive Function and Ageing Study (1999) Informal caregiving for frail older people at home and in long-term care institutions: who are the key supporters?, *Health and Social Care in the Community*, 7 (6): 434–44.

Roberts, E. (1984) *A Woman's Place: An Oral History of Working-class Women 1890–1940*. Oxford: Basil Blackwell.

Roberts, E. (1995) *Women and Families: An Oral History, 1940–1970*. Oxford: Blackwell.

Rodin, J. and Langer, E. (1980) Aging labels: the decline of control and the fall of self-esteem, *Journal of Social Issues*, 36: 12–29.

Rose, A. (1965) A current theoretical issue in social gerontology. In Rose, A. and Petersen, W. A. (eds) *Older People and their Social World*, Philadelphia, Pennsylvania: F.A. Davis Company.

Rowe, J. W. and Kahn, R. L. (1997) Successful aging, *Gerontologist*, 37 (4): 433–40.

Runciman, W. G. (1966) *Relative Deprivation and Social Justice*. London: Routledge and Kegan Paul.

Ruta, D. A., Garratt, A. M., Leng, M., Russell, I. T. and MacDonald, L. M. (1994) A new approach to the measurement of quality of life: the Patient-Generated Index. *Medical Care*, 32 (11): 1109–26.

Ryff, C. D. and Marshall, V. W. (1999) *The Self and Society in Ageing Processes*. New York: Springer.

Sarkisian, C. A., Hays, R. D., Berry, S. H. and Mangione, C. M. (2001) Expectations regarding aging among older adults and physicians who care for older adults, *Medical Care*, 39 (9): 1025–36.

Sawchuk, K. A. (1995) From gloom to boom: age, identity and target marketing. In Featherstone, M. and Wernick, A. (eds) *Images of Aging: Cultural Representations of Later Life*. London: Routledge.

Scambler, S., Victor, C. R., Bond, J. and Bowling, A. (2002) Promoting quality of life: preventing loneliness amongst older people. Paper presented to the XV World Congress of Sociology, 7–13 July, Brisbane.

Schutz, A. (1972) *The Phenomenology of the Social World*. London: Heinemann.

Schwartz, A. N. (1975) An observation on self esteem as the linchpin of quality of life for the aged, *Gerontologist*, 15: 470–2.

Schwartz, C. E. and Sprangers, M. A. G. (1999) Methodological approaches for assessing response shift in longitudinal health-related quality-of-life research, *Social Science and Medicine*, 48 (11): 1531–48.

Seligman, M. E. P. (1992) *Helplessness*. New York: W. H. Freeman.

Semmence, J., White, A., Wilkie-Jones, C., Butt, N. and Brown, S. (2000) *Family Resources Survey: Great Britain 1998–99*. London: The Stationery Office.

Shanas, E., Townsend, P., Wedderburn, D. *et al.* (1968) *Old People in Three Industrial Societies*. London: Routledge and Kegan.

Sheldon, J. H. (1948) *The Social Medicine of Old Age*. London: Oxford University Press.

Sheldrake, P. (1992) *Spirituality and History: Questions of Interpretation and Method*. New York: Crossroads.

Sidell, M. (1995) *Health in Old Age: Myth, Mystery and Management*. Buckingham: Open University Press.

Skucha, J. and Bernard, M. (2000) 'Women's work' and the transition to retirement. In Bernard, M., Phillips, J., Machin, L. and Harding Davies, V. (eds) *Women Ageing: Changing Identities, Challenging Myths*. London: Routledge.

Slater, R. (1995) *The Psychology of Growing Old: Looking Forward*. Buckingham: Open University Press.

Steptoe, A., Sutcliffe, I., Allen, B. and Coombes, C. (1991) Satisfaction with communication, medical knowledge, and coping style in patients with metastatic cancer, *Social Science and Medicine*, 32 (6): 627–32.

Stevens, N. (2001) Combating loneliness: a friendship enrichment programme for older women, *Ageing and Society*, 21 (2): 183–202.

Sugarman, L. (1986) *Life-span Development: Concepts, Theories and Interventions*. London: Methuen.

Tamke, S. S. (1978) Human values and aging: the perspective of the Victorian nursery. In Spicker, S. F., Woodward, K. M. and Van Tassel, D. D. (eds) *Aging and the Elderly: Humanistic Perspectives in Gerontology*. Atlantic Islands, New Jersey: Humanities Press.

Taylor, C. (1989) *Sources of the Self: The Making of the Modern Identity*. Cambridge: Cambridge University Press.

Taylor, R. C. and Ford, E. G. (1983) The elderly at risk: a critical examination of commonly identified risk groups, *Journal of the Royal College of General Practitioners*, 33: 699–705.

Thompson, P. (1992) I don't feel old: subjective ageing and the search for meaning in later life, *Ageing and Society*, 12: 23–47.

Thompson, P., Itzin, C. and Abendstern, M. (1991) *I Don't Feel Old. Understanding the Experience of Later Life*. Oxford: Oxford University Press.

Tobin, S. S. and Liebermann, M. A. (1976) *Last Home for the Aged: Critical Implications of Institutionalisation*. San Francisco, California: Jossey-Bass.

Tobin, S. S. and Neugarten, B. L. (1961) Life satisfaction and social interaction in the aging, *Journal of Gerontology*, 16: 344–6.

Torrance, G. W. (1986) Measurement of health state utilities for economic appraisal. A review, *Journal of Health Economics*, 5: 1–30.

Townsend, P. (1957) *The Family Life of Old People*. London: Routledge and Kegan.

Townsend, P. (1963) *The Family Life of Old People*, abridged edn. Middlesex: Penguin Books.

Townsend, P. (1964) *The Last Refuge: A Survey of Residential Institutions and Homes for the Aged in England and Wales*, abridged edn. London: Routledge and Kegan Paul.

Townsend, P. (ed.) (1970) *The Concept of Poverty*. London: Heinemann.

Townsend, P. (1973a) Isolation and loneliness in the aged. In Weiss, R. (ed.) *Loneliness: The Experience of Emotional and Social Isolation*, Cambridge, Massachusetts: The MIT Press.

Townsend, P. (1973b) *The Social Minority*. London: Allen Lane.

Townsend, P. (1979) *Poverty in the United Kingdom: A Survey of Household Resources and Standards of Living*. Harmondsworth: Penguin.

Townsend, P. (1981) The structured dependency of the elderly: a creation of social policy in the twentieth century, *Ageing and Society*, 1: 5–28.

Townsend, P. (1991) The social and economic hardship of elderly people in London: new evidence from a survey and a discussion of the influence of social policy upon current trends, *Generations Bulletin of the British Society of Gerontology*, 9: 10–30.

Townsend, P. and Tunstall, S. (1968) Isolation, desolation and loneliness. In Shanas, E., Townsend, P., Wedderburn, D. *et al.* (eds) *Old People in Three Industrial Societies*. London: Routledge and Kegan.

Townsend, P. and Wedderburn, D. (1965) *The Aged in the Welfare State*. London: Bell & Sons.

Tunstall, J. (1966) *Old and Alone. A Sociological Study of Old People*. London: Routledge and Kegan.

Victor, C., Scambler, S., Bond, J. and Bowling, A. (2000) Being alone in later life: loneliness, social isolation and living alone. *Reviews in Clinical Gerontology*, 10: 407–17.

Victor, C. R., Scambler, S. J., Bond, J. and Bowling, A. (2004) Older people's experiences of loneliness in the UK: does gender matter?, *Social Policy and Society* (in press).

Victor, C. R., Scambler, S. J., Shah, S. *et al.* (2002) Has loneliness amongst older people increased? An investigation into variations between cohorts, *Ageing and Society*, 22 (5): 585–97.

Wagner, G. (1988) *Residential Care: A Positive Choice*. London: HMSO.

Walker, A. (1980) The social creation of poverty and dependency in old age, *Journal of Social Policy*, 9: 59–75.

Walker, A. (1981) Towards a political economy of old age, *Ageing and Society*, 1: 73–94.

Walker, A. (1993) Poverty and inequality in old age. In Bond, J., Coleman, P. and Peace, S. (eds) *Ageing in Society. An Introduction to Social Gerontology*, 2nd edn. London: Sage Publications.

Walker, A. (2000) Public policy and the construction of old age in Europe, *Gerontologist*, 40 (3): 304–8.

Walker, A. and Taylor, P. (1993) Ageism versus productive aging: the challenge of age discrimination in the labor market. In Bass, S. A., Caro, F. G. and Chen, Y.-P. (eds) *Achieving a Productive Aging Society*. Westport, Connecticut: Auburn House.

Waterworth, S. and Luker, K. (1990) Reluctant collaborators: do patients want to be involved in decisions concerning care?, *Journal of Advanced Nursing*, 15: 971–6.

Wenger, G. C. (1984) *The Supportive Network: Coping with Old Age*. London: George Allen and Unwin.

Wenger, G. C. (1990) Change and adaptation in informal support networks of elderly people in Wales 1979–1987, *Journal of Aging Studies*, 4 (4): 375–89.

Wenger, G. C. (1992) *Help in Old Age – Facing up to Change. A Longitudinal Network Study*. Institute of Human Ageing Occasional Papers 5. Liverpool: Liverpool University Press.

Wenger, G. C. (1996) Social networks and gerontology, *Reviews in Clinical Gerontology*, 6: 285–93.

Wenger, G. C., Davies, R., Shahtahmasebi, S. and Scott, A. (1996) Social isolation and loneliness in old age: review and model refinement, *Ageing and Society*, 16 (3): 333–58.

Wenger, G. C. and Jerrome, D. (1999) Change and stability in confidant relationships: findings the Bangor Longitudinal Study of Ageing, *Journal of Aging Studies*, 13 (3): 269–94.

WHO (World Health Organization) (1992) *ICD:10 International Statistical Classification of Diseases and Related Health Problems*, 10th edn. Geneva: World Health Organization.

Wilkin, D. and Hughes, B. (1987) Residential care of elderly people: the consumers' views, *Ageing and Society*, 7: 175–201.

Willcocks, D., Peace, S. and Kellaher, L. (1987) *Private Lives in Public Places: A Research-based Critique of Residential Life in Local Authority Old People's Homes*. London: Tavistock.

Williams, R. (1990) *A Protestant Legacy. Attitudes to Death and Illness among Older Aberdonians*. New York: Oxford University Press.

Williams, R. G. A. (1983) Concepts of health: an analysis of lay logic, *Sociology*, 17: 185–205.

Wilson, G. (1995) A postmodern approach to structured dependency theory, *Journal of Social Policy*, 26 (3): 341–50.

Young, M. and Willmott, P. (1957) *Family and Kinship in East London*. London: Routledge and Kegan Paul.

Zautra, A. and Hempel, A. (1984) Subjective well-being and physical health: a narrative literature review with suggestions for future research, *International Journal of Aging and Human Development*, 19: 95–110.

Index

Page numbers in *italics* refer to figures and tables.

SOCIAL THEORY, SOCIAL POLICY AND AGEING
A Critical Introduction

Carroll Estes, Simon Biggs and Chris Phillipson

In this important new book, three leading social theorists of old age present a critical review of key theoretical developments and issues influencing the study of adult ageing. The authors explore contemporary trends in social policy drawing on the experience of ageing in the USA, Europe and an increasingly global environment.

Particular attention is given to feminist perspectives on ageing, ethics and bio-medicine, successful and productive ageing, globalization and migration and the politics of ageing. Consideration is given in each case to the interaction between structural influences on social ageing and the experience of age and identity. The work ends with a manifesto for social theory, social policy and social change.

Social Theory, Social Policy and Ageing will be valuable reading for advanced students and practitioners taking courses in social theory, the sociology of old age and social gerontology.

0 335 20906 8 (Paperback)   0 335 20907 6 (Hardback)

GENDER AND AGEING
Changing Roles and Relationships

Sara Arber, Kate Davidson and Jay Ginn (Eds.)

This book is a follow-up to Arber and Ginn's award winning *Connecting Gender and Ageing* (1995). It contains original chapters from eminent writers on gender and ageing, addressing newly emergent areas within gender and ageing, including gender identity and masculinity in later life.

Early work on gender and ageing was dominated by a focus on older women. The present collection breaks with this tradition by emphasizing changing gender roles and relationships, gender identity and an examination of masculinities in midlife and later life. A theme running through the book is the need to reconceptualize partnership status, in order to understand the implications of both widowhood and divorce for older women and men, as well as new forms of relationships, such as Living Apart Together (LAT-relationships). There is also an underlying focus on how socio-economic circumstances influence the experiences of ageing and the ways transitions are negotiated.

Written with undergraduate students and researchers in mind, *Gender and Ageing* will be an invaluable text for those studying social gerontology, sociology of later life, gender studies, health and community care and social policy.

Contents

192pp   0335 21319 7 (Paperback)   0335 21320 0 (Hardback)